Lecture Notes
Urology

John Blandy
CBE, MA, DM, MCh, FRCS, FACS, (Hon), FRCSI
Emeritus Professor of Urology
University of London
London Hospital Medical College
London

Amir Kaisary
MA, ChM, FRCS
Consultant Urologist
The Royal Free Hospital
London

Sixth Edition

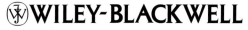
WILEY-BLACKWELL

A John Wiley & Sons, Ltd., Publication

This edition first published 2009, © by John Blandy and Amir Kaisary
Previous editions: 1976, 1977, 1982, 1989, 1998

Blackwell Publishing was acquired by John Wiley & Sons in February 2007.
Blackwell's publishing program has been merged with Wiley's global Scientific, Technical and Medical business to form Wiley-Blackwell.

Registered office: John Wiley & Sons Ltd, The Atrium, Southern Gate, Chichester, West Sussex, PO19 8SQ, UK

Editorial offices: 9600 Garsington Road, Oxford, OX4 2DQ, UK
The Atrium, Southern Gate, Chichester, West Sussex, PO19 8SQ, UK
111 River Street, Hoboken, NJ 07030-5774, USA

For details of our global editorial offices, for customer services and for information about how to apply for permission to reuse the copyright material in this book please see our website at www.wiley.com/wiley-blackwell

Library of Congress Cataloging-in-Publication Data

Blandy, John P. (John Peter), 1927-
  Lecture notes. Urology / John Blandy, Amir Kaisary. – 6th ed.
    p. ; cm.
  Includes index.
  Rev. ed. of: Lecture notes on urology / John Blandy. 5th ed. 1998.
  ISBN 978-1-4051-2270-2
1. Urinary organs–Diseases–Outlines, syllabi, etc.   2. Urology–Outlines, syllabi, etc.   I. Kaisary, Amir V.
II. Blandy, John P. (John Peter), 1927- Lecture notes on urology.   III. Title.   IV. Title:
Urology.
  [DNLM: 1. Urologic Diseases. WJ 140 B642L 2009]
  RC900.5.B53 2009
  616.6–dc22   2009013376

A catalogue record for this book is available from the British Library.

Set in 8/12pt Stone Serif by Aptara® Inc., New Delhi, India
Printed in Singapore

1   2009

Lecture Notes: Urology

Contents

Preface

More than 30 years ago, this book started as a set of brief notes mimeographed for medical students on the urology firm at The London Hospital. I hoped that students might find them helpful in understanding the patients and operations they saw on the wards and in the operating theatre. I believed that to understand the pathology of a condition was the key to understanding symptoms, signs and everything else. I also believed that pretty well every pathological process could be explained simply, that long-winded jargon was almost never needed, and in learning surgery as in most things, a spoonful of sugar helps the medicine go down.

Over 30 years, urology has seen extraordinary changes. New methods of imaging have transformed the precision of diagnosis. New techniques, especially laparoscopic surgery and the introduction of new lasers, have transformed operative surgery. My friend Amir Kaisary has worked hard to bring these notes up to date, without losing sight of their original intention, which was that students would find the subject interesting and yet has still managed to keep it clear and above all, we both hope, fun to read.

John Blandy

Acknowledgements

During preparation of this new edition we were both helped immensely by advice and contributions from many colleagues, for which we register our thanks. Special thanks also go to the Medical Illustration department at the Royal Free NHS Trust Hospital and Joint Royal Free and UCLH Medical School for the new artwork.

Anne and Karen, our wives, deserve a medal each for putting up with our moods during preparation of this book!

Further reading

It is now acknowledged that electronic communications ensure immediate access to sources of information without delay. You will note that there are no references listed at the end of chapters in this book. It is estimated that few months elapse between providing the text to publishers/printers and by the time the book is available on the market, few months have passed. This would inevitably make the material read not truly up to date. Continuous medical education (CME) would thus need the readers to get access to sources of education available electronically to keep you up to date. Useful sources are plentiful and here are some examples:

1 http://www.emedicine.com

This is an American-based website which is now internationally used. As a student you can register with this website for free. This will enable you to browse the information without having to pay for a subscription. This website gives an overview of the pathophysiology, epidemiology, clinical and radiographic findings and management options for most conditions.

2 www.pubmed.com or http://www.ncbi.nlm.nih.gov/sites/entrez/

PubMed is a service of the U.S. National Library of Medicine that includes over 18 million citations from MEDLINE and other life science journals for biomedical articles back to the 1950s. PubMed includes links to full text articles and other related resources. It is a useful tool where MEDLINE is not available to you or where you have not quite grasped how to use MEDLINE yet. It is user-friendly and provides links to articles that are relevant to your search. However, you will need an Athens password (and therefore subscription) to access most e-journals and articles.

3 http://wok.mimas.ac.uk/

Sign into the Web of Knowledge website in order to get to Web of Science. Again, you will need an Athens subscription of Web of Knowledge subscription. *Web of Science®* consists of seven databases containing information gathered from thousands of scholarly journals, books, book series, reports and more.

The three citation databases contain the references cited by authors of the articles. You can use these references to do cite reference searching. This type of search allows you to find articles that cite a previously published work.

Google scholar (http://scholar.google.co.uk) is a handy search tool because it will often return articles *and* books that have been published on the topic you are searching. It is deemed less academic compared to PubMed and is less useful if you are looking for recently published articles. However, with the power of Google as a search tool it will often find you active links to articles that can be accessed without a subscription.

Other valuable sites are UroSource Newsletters from European Association of Urology (EAU), Timely topics in Urology and web casts (info@ttmed.com and www.ttmed.com/urology), PeerView Press (webmaster@peerviewpress.com) and many more to find if you search.

This book gives you a lot and the initiative you take will give you more.

Amir V. Kaisary
John Blandy

Chapter 1

History and examination

Begin at the beginning: how old is your patient and what is his or her occupation? Do they smoke? Do they drink alcohol? Have they travelled in Africa or Indochina? Ask retired people about their previous occupation especially if there was any exposure to rubber, chemicals or plastics. Is there a family history of cancer? Women should be asked how many and how old are their children, and whether there was any complication during pregnancy or delivery that may have required catheterisation, which might have introduced infection.

What brings the patient to you? What were the first symptoms? When did they begin and how did they change as time went by? Let the patient do the talking – listening is the key to taking a history. Try to get a clear picture of the way the illness has developed over the years, and make sure you really understand just what is really bothering him or her right now. Never end your enquiry without asking whether the patient has noticed blood in the urine: haematuria is the single-most important symptom in the whole of urology, particularly if it is painless.

Your notes should be brief, but sufficiently clear that if you drop dead, another doctor can take up management of the case. No note is of any use if it cannot be read. If your handwriting is really bad, teach yourself to use a word processor. Put the date and name of the patient on every page. Always bear in mind that your notes are now available to the patient and may at any time be used as evidence in a court of law, so be polite about your patient and never be tempted to make a disparaging criticism of a professional colleague.

A drawing can save many words, so a sketch noting where the pain starts from and radiates to can be useful, together with a word or two to specify the type of pain, e.g. sharp, colicky or dull (Fig. 1.1). Avoid pretentious Greek or Latin terms unless they are clear and unambiguous. Dysuria can mean pain or difficulty or both: which do you really mean? Frequency is most simply expressed by writing down how often your patient voids by day and by night, e.g. D 6×, N 3×. Enuresis can be

Lecture Notes: Urology, 6th edition. By John Blandy and Amir Kaisary. Published 2009 by Blackwell Publishing. ISBN: 978-1-4051-2270-2.

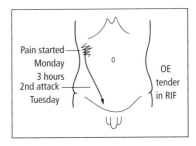

Figure 1.1 A sketch showing the main features in a patient with right ureteric colic.

ambiguous: if you mean the patient wets the bed, why not say so?

An exception is the term *haematuria*. It matters not whether the blood has been seen by the patient or found in a dipstick test, nor whether it is well mixed or appears at the beginning or the end of the stream: any kind of blood in the urine demands thorough investigation. Blood trickling from the urethra between acts of urination is probably coming from the urethra, but it still needs investigation.

Previous history

Ask about rheumatism and arthritis for which analgesics may have been taken: analgesic nephropathy is surprisingly common and seldom suspected unless you ask about the consumption of painkilling tablets.

Students often feel awkward when asking about venereal disease. In times past, men were usually secretly flattered at the suggestion that they might have been a Don Juan when young: today, one must be aware of the possibility of acquired immune deficiency syndrome (AIDS).

Do not waste time. As you listen to the patient it may be obvious that certain investigations are going to be needed. Unobtrusively filling in the relevant forms will not stop you from listening politely but will save time, and more importantly, may prevent you from writing down too much. Listening is far more important than writing.

Physical examination

Physical examination begins as the patient comes into the room. Does the patient look ill? Has the patient obviously lost weight? Does the gait suggest pain, Parkinsonism or ankylosing spondylitis? Is there that faint whiff of urine that suggests uraemia, or the ammoniacal reek of wet trousers?

To rise to shake your patient's hand is not mere politeness: it gives useful information. Whatever your specialty, never forget that you are a doctor first and your concern is for the patient as a whole. In an ideal world, where no doctor was ever pushed for time and no patient ever in a hurry to

get back to work or children, you could spend all day over one case, getting to know your patient in depth and making a thorough examination of every system. Something approaching such a thorough clerking may indeed be necessary when admitting a patient to the ward, but in the outpatient clinic it would be cruelly slow and unfair to the others who are waiting.

In most patients who attend the urological clinic, you are looking for enlargement of a kidney or bladder, disorders in the inguinal region or genitalia, hypertension and signs in the pelvis that might be detected by vaginal or rectal examination.

Abdominal examination

Kidney

The traditional physical signs of an enlarged kidney (Fig. 1.2) are:
• a rounded lump in the loin, bimanually palpable, moving on respiration;
• you can get your hand between the lump and the edge of the costal margin; and
• there is said to be a band of resonance in front of the kidney due to gas in the colon (Fig. 1.3).

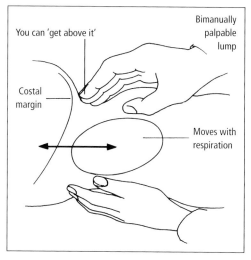

Figure 1.2 Physical signs of an enlarged kidney.

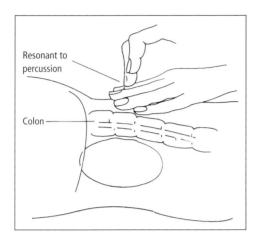

Figure 1.3 There is often a band of resonance in front of the kidney from gas in the colon.

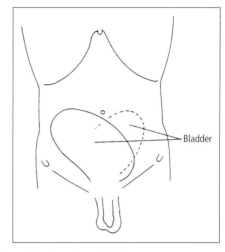

Figure 1.5 An enlarged bladder may go to one or other side.

None of these physical signs is trustworthy: on the right side the supposed 'kidney' may turn out to be the gall bladder or liver, and on the left it may prove to be the spleen, even though you think you can slide your hand between the lump and the costal margin. A large mass may arise from or displace the colon.

Bladder

An enlarged bladder (Figs. 1.4 and 1.5) may be equally misleading. One expects to find:

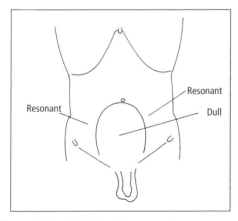

Figure 1.4 The bladder is dull to percussion.

- a rounded swelling arising out of the pelvis; and
- dull to percussion.

In practice, a floppy, over-distended bladder may be so soft that it is difficult to feel, and the bladder does not always rise up in the midline as expected, but is often more to one side than the other. The infallible sign is that the swelling goes away if you let the urine out with a catheter. Do not forget that an enlarged uterus arising from the pelvis could mimic a full, tense bladder.

Groin

Examination of the inguinal regions is concerned with three hernial orifices on each side (Fig. 1.6). Each must be felt with the patient standing up, lying down and coughing.

- An indirect inguinal hernia emerges lateral to the inferior epigastric vessels and slides down the inguinal canal to the scrotum.
- A direct inguinal hernia emerges medial to the inferior epigastric vessels, and seldom enters the scrotum.

Remember that direct and indirect inguinal herniae may be present in the same patient, with the two sacs emerging like a pair of trousers on either side of the inferior epigastric vessels (Fig. 1.7).

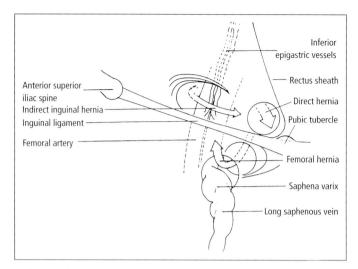

Figure 1.6 Landmarks for groin hernias.

• A femoral hernia pushes out below the inguinal ligament, medial to the femoral vein and then bulges up and out through the gap in the deep fascia where the saphenous vein joins the femoral vein. The sac has a narrow neck, and is always surrounded by a layer upon layer of fat like an onion, so that a cough impulse can be difficult to feel. A femoral hernia is mimicked by a saphena varix, the dilated upper end of the saphenous vein, but this has a cough thrill which runs down the saphenous vein, and the lump disappears when the patient lies down. If you help the patient to assume the sartorius position (hip flexion and lateral rotation), assessment of a possible femoral hernia can be made easier.

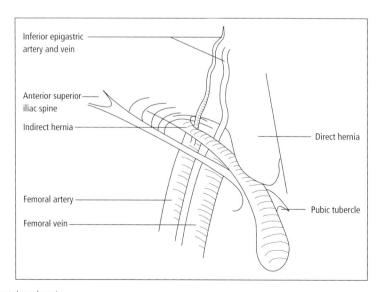

Figure 1.7 Pantaloon hernia.

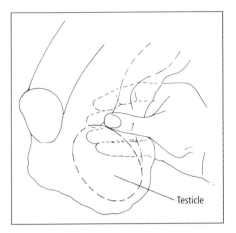

Figure 1.8 Lump in the scrotum: can you get above it?

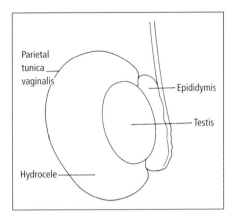

Figure 1.10 Hydroceles lie in front of the testis and tend to surround it.

The scrotum and its contents

The term 'testicle' includes testis and epididymis. When examining the scrotum, carry out the following simple steps:
• Can you 'get above' the swelling? If you can, it must be scrotal (Fig. 1.8).
• Is the lump fluctuant? Verify this by testing in two planes (Fig. 1.9). If it is fluctuant, then:
  If it is in front or around the testis, it is likely to be a hydrocele – fluid in the sac of the tunica vaginalis (Fig. 1.10); and
  If it is separate or behind the testis, it is likely to be a collection of cysts of the epididymis (Fig. 1.11).

• Can you shine a light through it? (An empty cylinder makes it easier to be sure of this in a well-lit room (Fig. 1.12).) If light does not shine through the swelling, either the wall of the swelling is thickened, or it contains not innocent clear fluid, but pus, blood or cancer.
• If the lump is not fluctuant, i.e. is solid, decide whether it is arising from the testis or the epididymis. A solid lump arising from the testis is cancer until proved otherwise (Fig. 1.13). A solid lump arising from the epididymis is usually benign, but calls for further investigation (Fig. 1.14).

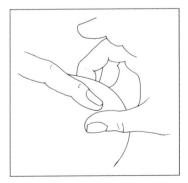

Figure 1.9 Lump in the scrotum: check whether it is solid or fluctuant. Determine fluctuation in two planes.

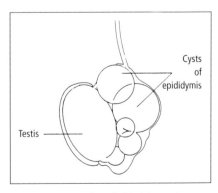

Figure 1.11 Cystic swellings behind the testis are cysts of the epididymis.

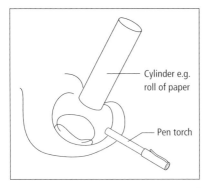

Figure 1.12 To see if light shines through a swelling, it helps to use a cylinder, e.g. one made from a rolled-up paper.

The spermatic cord

- *Varicocele:* The veins draining the testicle may become varicose and distended, feeling like a 'bag of worms', and there is a cough impulse (Fig. 1.15). (Like you, neither of us has ever actually felt a bag of worms, but we both know what it would feel like.)
- *Vas deferens:* The vas deferens lies posterior to the spermatic cord. If the vas is inflamed or has been operated on, e.g. by vasectomy, one may feel nodules along its course. Multiple knotty swellings are typical of tuberculosis (Fig. 1.16) and inflammatory swellings in the cord are seen in the tropical conditions of schistosomiasis and filariasis.

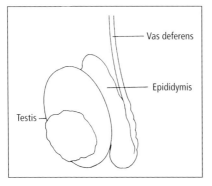

Figure 1.13 A solid swelling in the testis is a cancer until proved otherwise.

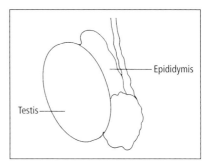

Figure 1.14 Solid swellings in the epididymis are usually inflammatory.

- *Encysted hydrocele of the cord:* When the testis descent in the scrotum is complete, the processus vaginalis closes completely forming a fibrous strand. If the closure happens proximally and distally only, this leaves a cystic structure within the spermatic cord which is mobile with it.

Rectal examination

One may perform a rectal examination in either sex in the supine, knee–elbow or left lateral position. Explain to your patient, what you are going

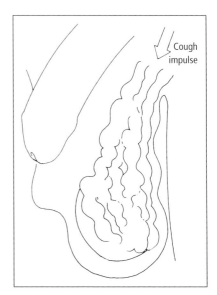

Figure 1.15 Varicocele: enlarged testicular veins. There is a cough impulse and the swelling disappears when the patient lies down.

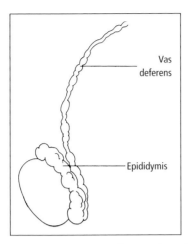

Figure 1.16 Multiple knotty swellings in the epididymis and a 'beaded' are highly suggestive of tuberculosis.

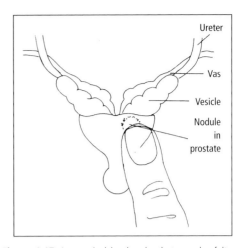

Figure 1.17 Anatomical landmarks that may be felt per rectum.

to do and ask his or her permission to do so. Always introduce your finger slowly and gently to allow the sphincter to relax (everyone knows the need to pass a constipated stool slowly). Once inside the rectum:
• Feel the wall of the rectum carefully – you will sometimes detect an entirely unexpected cancer of the rectum.

• Feel the prostate carefully for hardness or nodules which may mean cancer (Fig. 1.17). Even if it feels normal, try to estimate its diameters. If the prostate is tender on light palpation, it may be the site of inflammation.

Mistakes are easy to make when performing a rectal examination, but the worst mistake is not to do one at all.

Chapter 2

Investigations

Testing the urine

For centuries the doctor has learnt much from the urine: in times past, the doctor would look at it, measure it, smell it and even taste it. Today, he or she need not taste it. Infected urine usually stinks, and is always cloudy. Crystal clear urine is never infected. On many occasions a diagnosis may be made by having the patient simply record the time and volume of urine passed during 24 hours – the voiding diary or urine output chart (Fig. 2.1).

Office tests of the urine

pH

Indicator dyes impregnated on a paper strip measure pH sufficiently accurately for most purposes. Very acid urine should make you suspect uric acid stones. Very alkaline urine suggests infection with a microorganism that splits urea, e.g. *Proteus mirabilis*.

Protein

• Paper strips impregnated with tetrabromophenol normally turn blue in the pH range found in normal urine. Protein makes the colour yellowish. The dye is an indicator, and is therefore not reliable when the urine is very acid or very alkaline.

• A more reliable test for protein is to add a drop of 25% salicylsulphonic acid: this precipitates protein as a cloud unless the urine is exceptionally dilute.

• Boiling the urine precipitates a cloud, which persists when you add a drop of a dilute acid. If the cloud disappears, it was due to phosphates.

• When it is essential to know whether the quantity of protein in the urine is significant, collect the urine over 24 hours and have the protein measured quantitatively in the laboratory: more than 150 mg protein per 24 hours is abnormal and requires further investigation.

7.30 am	300 cc	Tuesday
8.15 "	150 cc	
11.10 "	100 cc	
12.35 pm	150 cc	
2.00 "	150 cc	
4.30 "	150 cc	
6.30 "	175 cc	
8.00 "	175 cc	
11.00 "	150 cc	
7.00 am	250 cc	Wednesday

Figure 2.1 Voiding diary or fluid output chart.

Lecture Notes: Urology, 6th edition. By John Blandy and Amir Kaisary. Published 2009 by Blackwell Publishing. ISBN: 978-1-4051-2270-2.

Glucose

• Paper strips are impregnated with potassium iodide and two enzymes: glucose oxidase converts glucose to gluconic acid and hydrogen peroxide; peroxidase then catalyses a reaction between hydrogen peroxide and potassium iodide to give a green–brown colour.

• If paper strips are unavailable, boil the urine with Fehling's or Benedict's solution. Glucose and other reducing substances throw down an orange precipitate of copper.

Blood in the urine

• Commercial stick tests for haematuria rely on the oxidation of tetramethylbenzidine by cumene peroxidase, which is catalysed by haemoglobin to give a green–blue colour, i.e. you are detecting free haemoglobin.

• If the test is positive, examine the urine under a microscope to confirm that red cells are present (see below).

The sensitivity of these stick tests is adjusted by the manufacturers to show a positive result when the amount of haemoglobin corresponds to about 10 red cells per high power field –twice the number found in normal urine – so a positive stick test always demands a thorough investigation. Remember that false-positive tests may occur if the glass container has been contaminated with povidone-iodine or has been cleaned with a bleaching agent such as hypochlorite.

Infection

Two stick tests for infection are available:
• based on bacterial conversion of nitrate to nitrite; and
• detection of leucocytes by leucocyte esterase activity.
In practice they are of limited use.

Bladder tumour antigen

The Bard bladder tumour antigen (BTA) test is based on the fact that bladder tumours break down the basement membrane, and liberate a protein – BTA – that can be detected by latex particles coated with human immunoglobulin G. The test strip produces a yellow band if positive, green if negative.

Microscopic examination of the urine

Blood

Put a drop of urine on a slide and cover with a cover slip. To find more than five red cells per high power field is abnormal.

Pus

A similar drop of urine will show more than five white cells per high power field if there is infection. When the pus cells come from the kidney, they have a characteristic glittering appearance. A Gram stain of the centrifuged deposit may identify which bacteria are present.

Casts

Casts are the squeezed-out contents of the collecting tubules of the kidney. When they are made of protein they are clear (hyaline): when made of red or white cells they are granular (Fig. 2.2).

Crystals

In cool urine there are always some crystals of triple phosphate and calcium oxalate. The hexagonal plates of cystine give away the diagnosis of cystinuria. Uric acid crystals are especially common in acid urine (Fig. 2.3).

Mycobacterium tuberculosis

The centrifuged urine is stained with auramine and examined under ultraviolet light: the mycobacteria shine as bright yellow dots.

Cancer cells

The urine is fixed with a roughly equal volume of 10% formalin and sent to the laboratory. There it

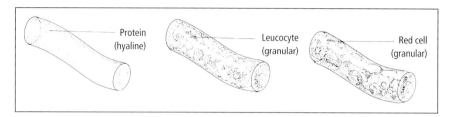

Figure 2.2 Casts in the urine.

is centrifuged: the deposit is made into a smear and stained with methylene blue (Papanicolaou's method; Fig. 2.4). Anaplastic tumour cells are larger and have bigger nuclei than normal urothelium. Note common sources of error:
• False-negatives may occur if the tumour is well differentiated when the shed cells are hardly different from normal urothelium.

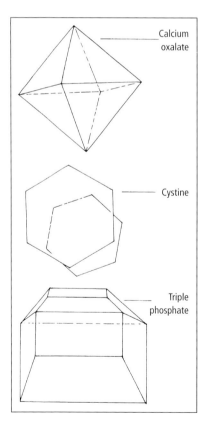

Figure 2.3 Crystals in the urine.

• False-positives occur if part of the urothelium is undergoing mitosis in course of healing after some recent injury, e.g. from the passage of a stone.

Schistosoma ova

The centrifuged deposit of urine may show the characteristic ova of Schistosoma. The different species have ova of characteristic shape (Fig. 2.5).

Culture of urine

Urine is an excellent culture medium and is easily contaminated from the wall of the urethra, prepuce or vulva, or by air-borne dust. At room temperature contaminants grow rapidly so that urine must either be plated out at once, or put in a refrigerator. A mistaken diagnosis of infection may be made if the urine is allowed to stand around at room temperature for a few hours before reaching the laboratory. The urine is obtained in three ways:
• By needle aspiration of the bladder. Any organisms found are abnormal.
• By catheterisation, but passing a catheter is uncomfortable and may introduce infection.
• By 'clean-catch' specimen or 'mid-stream urine'. Urine is mixed with a culture medium before incubation. Each organism gives rise to one colony, so a colony count shows how many bacteria were present in the urine. As a rule more than 50,000 (10^5) colonies/mL signifies infection, and anything less means contamination. Remember that these figures only apply to clean-voided urine. One easy way to make a colony-count is with a dip-slide (Fig. 2.6). Plastic slides coated with culture media are dipped in urine, drained off, placed in a sterile bottle and incubated. After 12 hours, a glance at

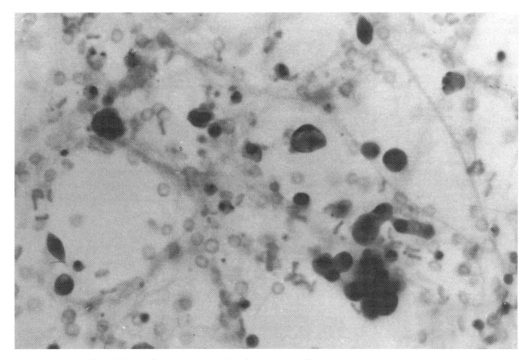

Figure 2.4 Centrifuged deposit from urine stained to show cancer cells.

the chart supplied with the slide shows whether there are more than 10^5 colonies or not.

Imaging the urinary tract

Plain abdominal radiograph ('scout film'; kidney, ureter and bladder (KUB) etc.)

Check adequacy of the film. It must include the bladder base and the prostate urethral region in order not to miss a urethral stone. Look at each film with four Ss in mind (Fig. 2.7):

• *Side:* Radiographers, being only human, sometimes put the wrong letter on the film. Always check that the soft tissue shadow of the liver is on the right side and the gastric air bubble on the left.

• *Skeleton:* Check the spine, ribs, hips and sacroiliac joints for bony metastases, the evidence of ankylosing spondylitis, or loss of joint space in the hips for which the patient might have taken

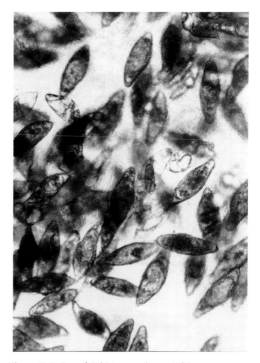

Figure 2.5 Ova of *Schistosoma haematobium.*

11

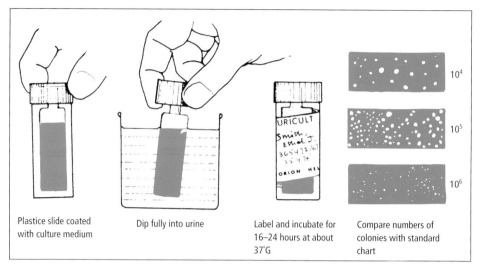

Plastice slide coated with culture medium

Dip fully into urine

Label and incubate for 16–24 hours at about 37°G

Compare numbers of colonies with standard chart

Figure 2.6 Dip-slide method of estimating colony count.

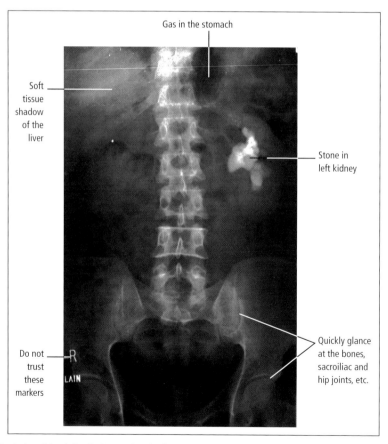

Gas in the stomach

Soft tissue shadow of the liver

Stone in left kidney

Do not trust these markers

Quickly glance at the bones, sacroiliac and hip joints, etc.

Figure 2.7 Check the plain abdominal X-ray for the four Ss: side, skeleton, soft tissues and stones.

analgesics and incurred the risk of analgesic nephropathy. In children with enuresis, careful examination of the lumbosacral spine is essential to exclude spina bifida defects.

• *Soft tissues:* In fat people the kidneys are surrounded by radiolucent fat which defines their outlines. A distended bladder or an enlarged uterus will fill the pelvis and displace the usual bowel gas shadows. In order to detect a large bladder residual volume, it is often helpful to obtain the film after voiding.

• *Stones:* Any radio-opaque shadow in the line of the urinary tract might be a stone. If it seems to be in the kidney, it should move up and down with the kidney during respiration. 'Stones' in the pelvis often turn out to be calcified fibroids or phleboliths. Only 60–70% of stones are dense enough to be visible on radiographs.

Intravenous urogram or pyelogram

This investigation allows good visualisation of the collecting systems and ureters. It is predominantly used to investigate haematuria and also to determine the ureteric anatomy. More recently its use in renal pain, ureteric colic and urinary stone disease has been replaced by computerised axial tomography/KUB (spiral CAT) studies.

Contrast media

Its high atomic number makes iodine relatively opaque to X-rays. Free ionic iodine is toxic, but when joined to benzoic acid it forms organic salts which can be given in large quantities, usually with safety. It does however have several drawbacks:

• *Chemical irritation:* Occasionally irritation of the vein results in flushing, nausea and vomiting, when the bolus of hypertonic contrast medium reaches the systemic circulation. These effects are not common and seldom serious. Chemical inflammation and necrosis of skin could result if the hypertonic solution is accidentally injected outside the vein. This is less of a concern now as the contrast media used are non-ionic and of low osmolarity.

• *Allergy:* True allergy to contrast medium is much more serious. It can range from a trivial urticarial rash which will vanish with an antihistamine, to life-threatening oedema of the glottis, trachea and bronchi, with widespread vasodilatation, hypotension and cardiac arrest. The allergen is the complete iodobenzoate molecule, not free iodine, so it is futile to perform skin tests with iodine. The reaction is not avoided by giving the first few millilitres of contrast slowly.

Millions of intravenous urograms (IVUs) are done every year, and fatal reactions occur only in 1:200,000. Patient anxiety increases the likelihood of a reaction thus quick reassurance to patients by the staff is helpful. Essential precautions are:

• Always enquire about even the most trivial previous reaction to contrast media.

• Be always ready for one. Never start to give intravenous contrast medium without first making sure for yourself that all the essentials for treating an allergic reaction are to hand and within reach of the X-ray table. There must be:
  • adrenaline;
  • hydrocortisone;
  • oxygen, with face-mask and airway;
  • a 'minitracheostomy' kit; and
  • a 'panic button' that will summon the cardiac arrest team.

Contrast medium in the kidney

Nephrogram

It takes 15–20 seconds for the contrast medium to reach the kidney. Contrast medium should be injected rapidly in order to ensure the bolus reaches the kidneys quickly. A film taken in the first 30 seconds will catch the contrast as it lies in the glomeruli and proximal tubules where water is being reabsorbed, so this, the 'immediate' or 'nephrogram' film, gives an image of the renal parenchyma (Fig. 2.8). Note that:

• When it is particularly important to obtain a good picture of the renal outline, e.g. when scarring or a tumour is suspected, then tomograms are taken during the nephrogram phase to eliminate unwanted shadows from gas in the bowel.

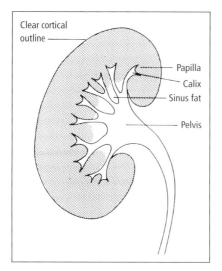

Figure 2.8 Nephrogram phase of IVU.

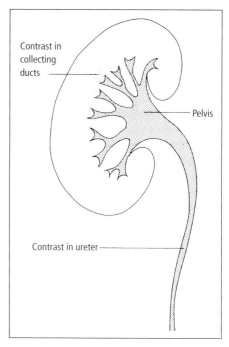

Figure 2.9 Pyelogram phase of IVU.

• In obstruction the filtrate cannot escape down the tubule, and so the nephrogram is denser and lasts longer. (With a stone blocking the ureter it is quite common to see the nephrogram persist for 24 hours or more.)

Pyelogram

In a normal patient the glomerular filtrate containing the contrast medium quickly reaches the calices and pelvis to give the pyelogram (Fig. 2.9). A film taken at 5 minutes will therefore show the relationships of the calices to the renal contour and many centres obtain this 'pyelogram' film in place of the 1-minute film in order to limit radiation exposure dose. The calices can be filled out by compressing the abdomen with a tight band to squeeze the ureters for the first 10–15 minutes. This compression is only applied if there are more of the following: evidence of obstruction, in children, and history of trauma, aneurism or recent abdominal surgery.

• A film taken just after releasing the band will then show the whole length of the ureter. If a portion of the ureter is shown poorly, obtaining oblique views often results in better visualisation.

• Later films are taken to show the contrast in the bladder (Fig. 2.10).

• The patient then empties the bladder, and if there is any question about the urethra, oblique films are taken during micturition to give a descending urethrogram. Afterwards a post-micturition film is taken which gives a rough idea of the volume of residual urine.

If one kidney is very small or scarred, most of the solute load has to be eliminated by the other one. In the small kidney the filtrate flows only slowly down the tubules, and in doing so becomes sufficiently concentrated to give a misleadingly clear image: never mistake a good image for good function.

Preparation for IVU studies

The obsolete practice still lingers of preparing patients for an IVU by depriving them of fluid for 6 hours or longer. This may give a slight increase in the concentration of contrast in the filtrate, and perhaps a marginal improvement in the image, but in a normal patient given the usual amount of contrast the improvement does not justify the

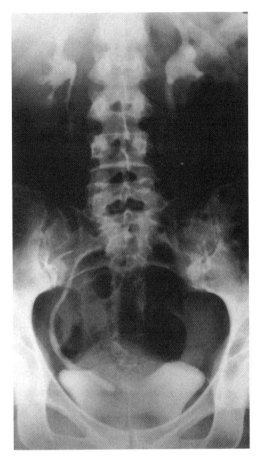

Figure 2.10 The upper tracts and bladder are shown in the 20-minute film of the IVU.

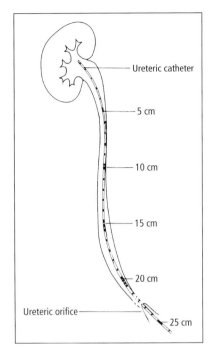

Figure 2.11 Retrograde pyelogram with a ureteric catheter.

discomfort to the patient. Not only is the practice usually futile, it can be dangerous:

• the period of starvation can be dangerous in diabetes; and

• in myeloma it may lead to anuria from protein blocking the tubules.

To postpone an IVU merely because the patient 'is not prepared' should not be accepted as an excuse. Always obtain a control film.

Retrograde urogram

A fine ureteric catheter is passed up the ureteric orifice through a cystoscope and contrast medium is injected to outline the ureter, pelvis and calices

(Fig. 2.11). A bulb-ended catheter jammed in the ureteric orifice allows dye injection up the whole length of the ureter (the ureterogram; Fig. 2.12) without possible leak back in the bladder. These retrograde studies are performed under X-ray control.

Antegrade or descending urogram

A fine needle is passed into the renal pelvis under X-ray or ultrasound control. A flexible guidewire is passed through the needle into the pelvis, the needle is withdrawn, and a cannula slipped over the guidewire into the pelvis to perform a percutaneous nephrostomy (Fig. 2.13). This is the first step in a whole range of percutaneous operations on the kidney. Contrast medium injected through the cannula will delineate the renal pelvis and ureter. The pressure inside the cannula can be measured at the same time in the course of investigating obstruction.

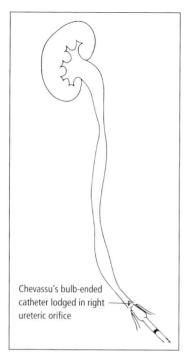

Chevassu's bulb-ended catheter lodged in right ureteric orifice

Figure 2.12 Retrograde ureteropyelogram using a bulb-ended catheter.

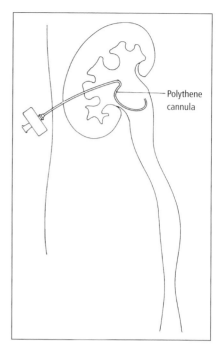

Polythene cannula

Figure 2.13 Percutaneous nephrostomy to obtain descending or antegrade pyelogram.

Cystogram

The image of the bladder in the standard IVU will usually show diverticula or large tumours of the bladder (Fig. 2.14). If the picture is not clear, or when it is necessary to rule out reflux from the bladder up the ureters, or in order to investigate incontinence, then the bladder is filled with contrast and screened while the patient passes urine. This is often combined with measurements of the pressure inside the bladder and the urine flow rate in a micturating cystometrogram.

Urethrography

In investigating strictures and other disorders of the urethra an ascending urethrogram is made by injecting contrast medium into the urethra with a small catheter. As opacification of the female urethra is technically difficult, this study is predominantly performed in men.

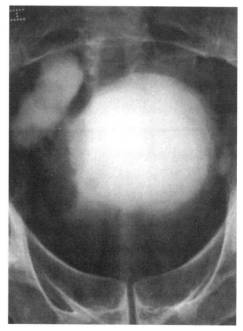

Figure 2.14 Cystogram image at the end of the IVU, in this case showing a diverticulum on the right side of the bladder.

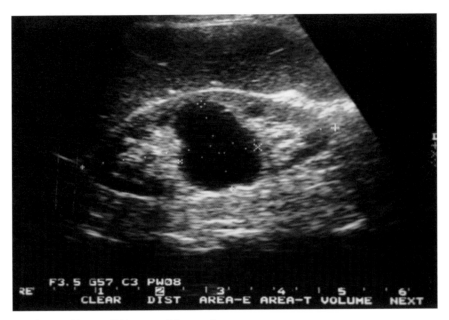

Figure 2.15 Ultrasound image of kidney containing a cyst.

Ultrasound

Ultrasonography is cheap, painless and uses no dangerous radiation. An AC current is applied to a piezoelectric crystal which then pulsates and produces a sound wave. The resulting wave penetrates soft tissues and is reflected by interfaces between tissues of different density, e.g. renal calices and parenchyma, or a renal cyst and parenchyma (Fig. 2.15). The returning echoes are received by the crystal which reverses the process. The sound is converted into an electrical impulse which is processed by a computer to give an image. Ultrasound images are more meaningful if you see them moving on a screen yourself. As images are obtained in a real-time mode, it is an excellent guide to interventional procedures, e.g. nephrostomy. It is the method of choice in paediatrics.

Transluminal ultrasound

By inserting a special probe into the rectum (transrectal ultrasound; TRUS), high-resolution images can be obtained of the prostate (Fig. 2.16). This allows geographically mapped guided prostate biopsies. Transvaginal ultrasound has been particularly valuable in the detection of urethral diverticula.

Angiography

A flexible guidewire is passed through a needle in the femoral artery over which a flexible cannula with a curved tip is slipped, and guided under X-ray control into the opening of the renal artery. Contrast is then injected into the renal artery or its branches to give an arteriogram (Fig. 2.17). This investigation can be of value in the diagnosis of trauma, stenosis of the renal artery and where the cause of haematuria proves to be particularly hard to discover. Similar studies are made when it is suspected that there may be extension of tumour into the vena cava (cavography; Fig. 2.18). The image of smaller vessels in the angiogram can be improved if overlying shadows of bone and bowel gas are removed: this can be done with a computer (Fig. 2.19) to give a digital subtraction angiogram. Renal venography has been largely replaced by ultrasonography or contrast-enhanced CAT or MRI. One remaining indication is the cannulation of

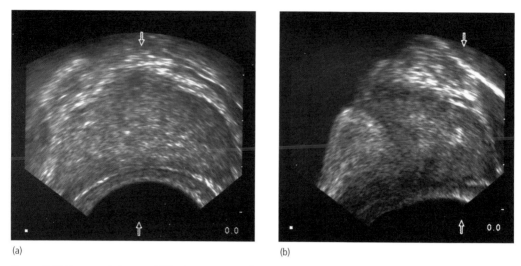

(a) (b)

Figure 2.16 Transrectal ultrasound (TRUS) examination of the prostate: (a) transverse and (b) longitudinal.

the gonadal veins with a view to embolisation in cases of scrotal varicocoeles.

Computed tomography

The CAT image is obtained by the computerised calculation of X-ray absorption after thousands of pencil thin beams of X-rays are transmitted through a patient as a rotating source whilst the patient moves through the source on a table (hence producing a 'spiral' data set. This technique provides exquisitely good spatial resolu-

tion but does involve a high radiation dose. It is the test of choice in urolithiasis, staging of renal cell carcinoma and the evaluation of renal tract

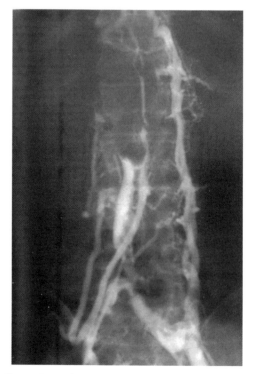

Figure 2.18 Inferior vena cavogram showing tumour in the vena cava.

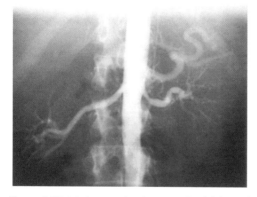

Figure 2.17 Arteriogram showing stenosis of left renal artery.

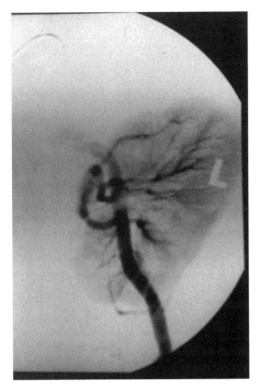

Figure 2.19 Subtraction angiogram of a renal transplant in the left iliac fossa.

trauma (dynamic CT scanning). It can be supplemented with contrast, e.g. intravenous dye injections (CAT/IVU combination) (see Fig. 2.20).

Magnetic resonance imaging

Atoms behave like gyroscopes whose axes are tilted by a strong magnetic field. When the field is turned off the gyroscopes whip back to their original position, and as they do so, give off a pulse of electromagnetic energy – magnetic resonance – which can be detected by a set of electronic sensors, mounted in a hoop and processed by computer to give an image (Fig. 2.21). This technique is becoming increasingly available and has the advantage of not involving irradiation or iodide contrast medium. Current indications for urological MRI include the local staging of pelvic urological cancers, assessing the degree of venous involvement

of a renal cell cancer and the detection of renal artery stenosis. Some centres use MRI routinely in patients with impaired renal function in whom the use of nephrotoxic contrast medium is inadvisable. Patients who have pacemakers and metal surgical devices are not suitable for this type of investigation.

Radio-isotope studies

Radionuclides are tagged on to various pharmaceuticals (often with very long names!) to create radiopharmaceuticals. These are administered to the patient to provide functional imaging, and in some cases quantification, of various bodily processes. The radionuclide decays, and as it does so, emits small packets of energy (usually gamma photons) which interact with the detector crystal on a gamma camera, to cause a small flash of light to be emitted. This flash of light is then converted into an electrical current and amplified by an array of photomultiplier tubes on the back of the crystal. The resulting current is then put through a range of electronic wizardry and a digital image is produced. The more radiopharmaceutical materials are taken up, the brighter the image.

Four radiopharmaceuticals are most commonly used in renal imaging:

1 ^{99m}Tc *benzoylmercaptoacetyltriglycerine* (more conveniently known as MAG3) is secreted by the proximal tubules into the tubular lumen.

2 ^{99m}Tc *diethylenetriamine pentaacetic acid* (DTPA) is excreted predominantly by glomerular filtration. Both of these agents are used for dynamic renography, which allows time activity curves to be produced (Fig. 2.22) that show how the kidneys handle the tracer and give a good idea of how well each kidney is functioning. The images also give valuable information about the anatomical appearance of the kidneys although in less detail than ultrasound or CAT. Better results in patients with poorer renal function are obtained from MAG3 than DTPA.

3 ^{99m}Tc *2,3 dimercaptosuccinic acid* (DMSA) is taken up and 'fixed' by the tissues of the proximal convoluted tubules. This radiopharmaceutical is not

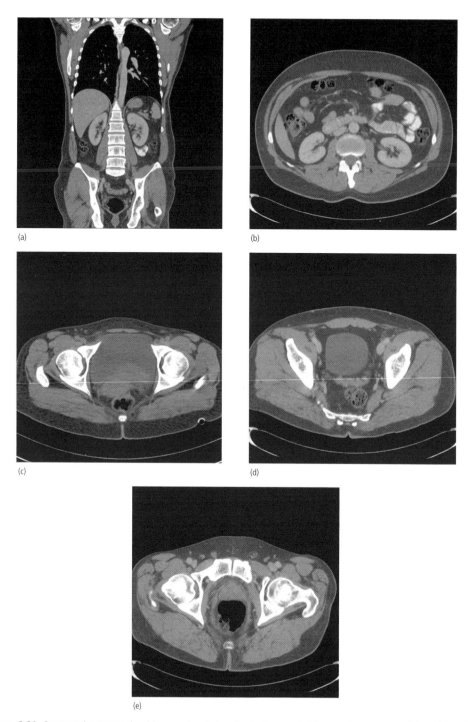

(a)

(b)

(c)

(d)

(e)

Figure 2.20 Computed tomography: (a) normal male longitudinal coronal; (b) normal transverse axial at kidney level; (c) normal female transverse axial at bladder and uterus level; (d) normal male transverse axial at bladder level; and (e) normal male transverse axial at prostate level.

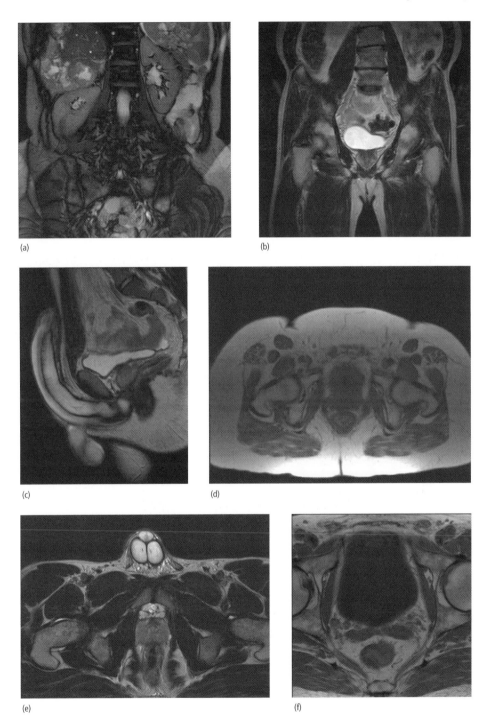

Figure 2.21 MRI scan: (a) normal upper abdomen; (b) normal pelvis; (c) lateral normal male pelvis; (d) transverse normal female pelvis; (e) transverse normal male pelvis at prostate level; and (f) transverse normal male pelvis at seminal vesicles level.

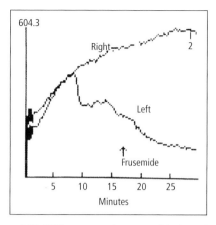

Figure 2.22 DTPA renogram in a case of hydronephrosis showing hold up of contrast on the right side, in spite of frusemide.

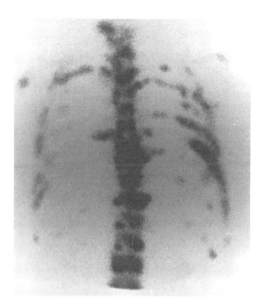

Figure 2.24 Bone scan in a man with carcinoma of the prostate with widespread metastases.

used for renography, but does provide important information about the renal cortex (e.g. detecting renal scars Fig. 2.23), locating ectopic kidneys and in evaluation of relative renal function (L:R ratios).
4 $^{51}Chromium\ EDTA$ is used to determine the glomerular filtration rate. This test involves only measurements of radioactivity in blood samples after intravenous injection of the radiopharmaceutical. No images are acquired.

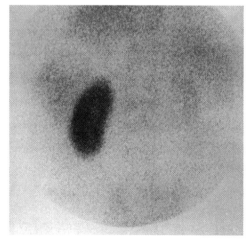

Figure 2.23 DMSA scan showing a normal right kidney but almost no uptake on the left, due to severe scarring.

Other nuclear medicine tests that are useful in urology include the bone scan. This is usually performed with ^{99m}Tc methylene diphosphonate (MDP) which is taken up wherever there is active bone turnover and gives rise to a 'hot spot'. It is not a very specific test but is extremely sensitive. The pattern of hot spots throughout the skeleton is important. Bony metastases often give rise to a random scatter throughout the axial skeleton and proximal long bones. This appearance is typical of prostate cancer (Fig. 2.24).

Positron emission tomography (PET) is a special type of isotope scan in which two high-energy gamma photons (180° apart) are emitted from each atomic disintegration. The isotopes used in the radiopharmaceuticals have short half lives (typically 10–60 minutes). The most commonly used radiopharmaceutical for PET imaging is ^{18}F fluoro-2 deoxyglucose (FDG). This is taken up by any cell which actively metabolises glucose. Cells which have more active metabolism (e.g. many cancers) will take up more than surrounding cells. These radiopharmaceuticals are detected by a PET scanner. Recent advances have made it possible to combine a PET scan with a conventional CAT scan. The patient undergoes a CAT scan immediately followed by a PET scan. The images from both scans can then be fused. This method of scanning beautifully combines functional imaging with high-resolution anatomical imaging so that pathology on a CAT scan effectively 'lights up'. This method is very useful in oncological imaging.

Chapter 3

The kidney: structure and function

Surgical relations of the kidney

Posterior relations

The kidneys are well protected, tucked in on either side of the spine.
- Behind each kidney is the lung, constantly moving up and down, so the inferior border of the kidney may lie anywhere between the 2nd and 4th lumbar transverse processes.
- The other posterior relations of the kidney are the 12th rib, diaphragm, quadratus lumborum and Psoas muscles (Fig. 3.1).
- The ilioinguinal and hypogastric nerves cross the quadratus lumborum muscle and are often injured in approaching the kidney from the loin.

Anterior relations: left

- The tail of the pancreas and the spleen lie in front of the left kidney and are easily injured at operation. The duodenojejunal flexure and descending colon also lie just in front of the left kidney, so indigestion or bowel distension is common when there is inflammation or obstruction of the kidney, and cancer of the kidney easily invades the adjacent bowel (Fig. 3.2a,b).

Lecture Notes: Urology, 6th edition. By John Blandy and Amir Kaisary. Published 2009 by Blackwell Publishing. ISBN: 978-1-4051-2270-2.

Anterior relations: right

- ascending colon;
- the second part of the duodenum; and
- common bile duct: it is not surprising that 'indigestion' often accompanies disorders of the right kidney (Fig. 3.3a,b)

Surgical approaches to the kidney

Posterior

Percutaneous nephrostomy

A needle passed into the renal pelvis goes through skin, latisimus dorsi, quadratus lumborum, perirenal fat and renal parenchyma. It is easy to understand how by mischance the needle may pierce the pleura, liver, duodenum or colon.

Twelfth rib approach

Most open operations on the kidney are performed through an incision along the bed of the 12th rib. Despite every precaution the pleura is often opened. The 11th and 12th subcostal nerves as well as the ilioinguinal and hypogastric nerves are always stretched and sometimes cut: postoperative pain is often severe and chest complications are common (Fig. 3.4).

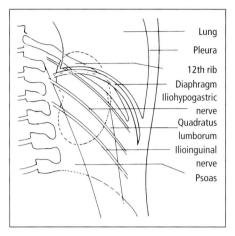

Figure 3.1 Posterior anatomical relations of the kidney.

Vertical lumbotomy

A vertical incision along the lateral border of sacrospinalis may free the attachments of the abdominal muscles. It gives limited access to the kidney but avoids much of the pain of the 12th rib approach (Fig. 3.5).

Thoracoabdominal incision

Very large cancers demand perfect exposure. The incision is carried through the bed of the 10th rib, across the pleura and into the abdomen. The lung and liver are retracted. The improved access to the inferior vena cava and aorta allows the surgeon to avoid and control bleeding and remove tumour that extends into the renal vein.

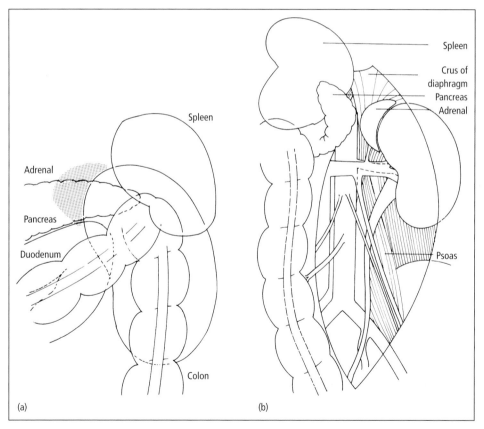

Figure 3.2 (a) Anatomical relations of the left kidney. (b) Left kidney and surrounding structures displayed at operation by reflecting the colon, spleen and tail of pancreas medially.

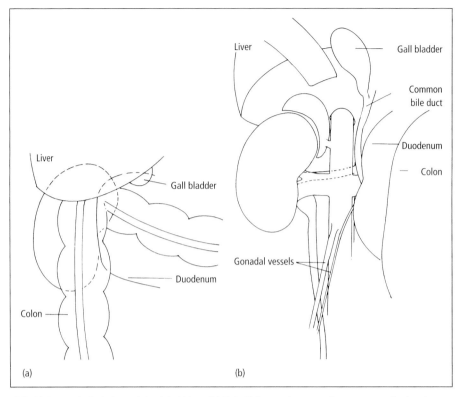

Figure 3.3 (a) Anatomical relations of the right kidney. (b) Right kidney and surrounding structures displayed at operation by reflecting the colon and duodenum medially.

Anterior

Minimal access surgery

Extraperitoneal
A balloon is passed though a cannula introduced into the perirenal fat. It is blown up to separate the peritoneum, duodenum and colon from the kidney and kept blown up long enough for bleeding to stop. When it is deflated, it leaves an empty space into which laparoscopic instruments may be introduced to carry out various operations on the kidney.

Transperitoneal
Carbon dioxide is introduced into the peritoneal cavity with a small cannula and then a number of 'ports' are made through which large cannulae are pushed into the gas-filled space. Through these other instruments are passed to reflect the colon and duodenum off the front of the kidney and allow the planned operation to take place.

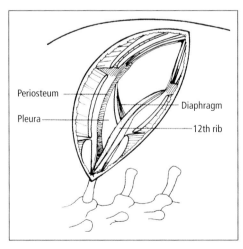

Figure 3.4 Twelfth rib bed approach to the right kidney.

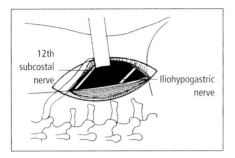

Figure 3.5 Vertical lumbotomy approach to the right kidney.

Conventional open surgery

With a large cancer of the kidney safety demands perfect exposure to control the renal artery and vein. The choice of either a transverse or midline incision is determined by the build of the patient (Figs. 3.6 and 3.7). The ascending colon, hepatic flexure and duodenum are reflected medially to give safe access to the right renal vessels (Fig. 3.8). On the left side reflection of the splenic flexure, descending colon and duodenojejunal flexure will give safe access to the left renal vessels (Fig. 3.9).

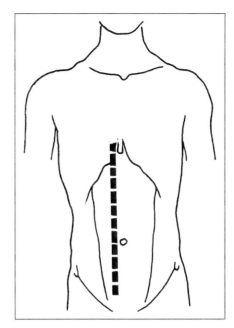

Figure 3.7 Transabdominal approach through vertical incision in a long thin patient.

Complications after renal surgery

The surgical relations of the kidney explain most of the common postoperative complications.

Pain

There is always postoperative pain on breathing and coughing. Postoperative pain can inhibit coughing and lead to atelectasis and infection in the empty lung segments. This is more common when the pleura has been opened or if part of the rib has had to be removed.

Pneumothorax

This may require aspiration or underwater drainage.

Ileus

Oedema or haematoma behind the bowel may lead to a period of abdominal distension and paralytic ileus.

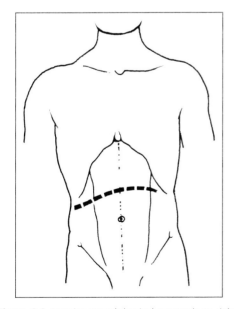

Figure 3.6 Anterior transabdominal approach to right kidney through a transverse incision.

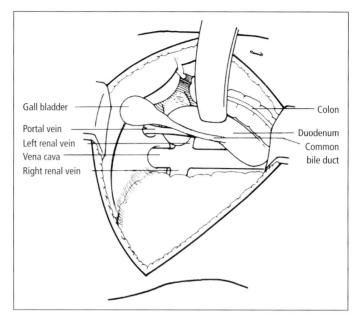

Figure 3.8 Operative exposure of right kidney: colon and duodenum reflected.

Structure of the kidney

Renal pyramid

The basic unit of the mammalian kidney is the pyramid. In porpoises the pyramids remain separate so that the kidney looks like a bunch of grapes. In most other mammals (including man) the porpoise arrangement is still seen in the foetus. In the adult, the dozen pyramids are squeezed together (Fig. 3.10). Each pyramid is like a bunch of flowers in a vase (Fig. 3.11), the blooms are the *glomeruli*,

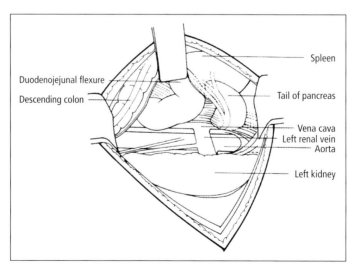

Figure 3.9 Operative exposure of left kidney: spleen, colon and duodenum reflected.

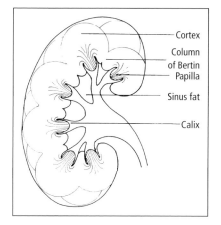

Figure 3.10 The kidney is formed of a collection of pyramids squeezed together: where they merge they form the columns of Bertin.

the stems the *collecting ducts* and the whole bunch, the *papilla*, sits in a vase, the *calix*.

Renal papilla

The collecting ducts open onto the papilla obliquely so that when pressure rises in the calix the ducts are closed as if by a valve (Fig. 3.12).

Children may be born with papillae that are fused together – *compound papillae*. These make the valve mechanism ineffective so that if the pressure in the pelvis rises, e.g., from *obstruction* or *reflux*, urine is forced into the renal parenchyma where it may cause inflammation and scarring (Fig. 3.13).

The collecting ducts gather the glomerular filtrate from the *nephrons* which are arranged like corn on the cob (Fig. 3.14). Each nephron has two parts: a filter, the *glomerulus*, and a processing plant, the *renal tubules*.

Glomerulus

The glomerulus is made of an arteriole, coiled like a ball of wool, which is invaginated into a hollow balloon – *Bowman's capsule* – whose stem drains into the *proximal tubule* (Fig. 3.15). The glomerular arteriole is very permeable, with an endothelium specially dimpled to increase its porosity. Its basement membrane is supported like filter paper on a grid formed by the *foot processes* of the epithelial cells of Bowman's capsule, which interlock like a zip-fastener (Fig. 3.16). The spaces between the zip are called *slit-pores* and their size has been measured using peroxidases of known molecular mass:

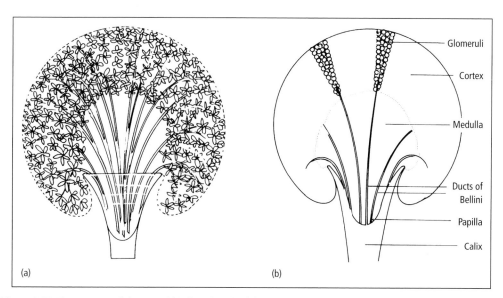

Figure 3.11 The structure of the pyramid is like a bunch of flowers in a vase.

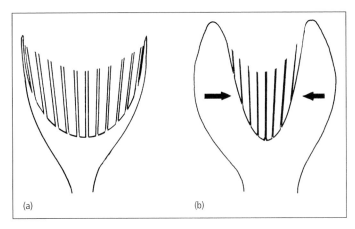

Figure 3.12 Valvular arrangement of a normal papilla.

those of molecular mass less than 40,000 can slip through: those above 160,000 get stuck.

Filtration is not merely a matter of the size of the molecule. The proteins of the basement membrane are negatively charged. They repel negatively charged molecules, e.g. albumen, but allow positively charged molecules of similar size to pass through. The pressure inside the glomerular arteriole is about 60 mm Hg. The *plasma oncotic pressure* is about 25 mm Hg, so that there is a *filtration pressure* of about 35 mm Hg. The pressure inside Bowman's capsule is about 10 mm Hg.

The arterioles of the glomeruli are 50 times more permeable than those of arterioles elsewhere, e.g. muscle, and they allow enormous volumes of fluid

to leak out. The whole plasma water is filtered every 30 minutes and the entire body water processed four times a day. The first task of the tubules is to recapture this huge amount of water.

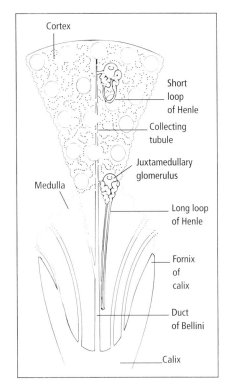

Figure 3.14 Nephrons arranged on their collecting tubule like corn on the cob.

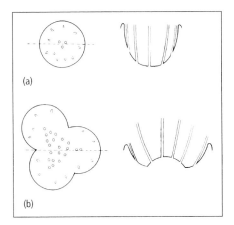

Figure 3.13 (a) Normal papilla and (b) compound papilla.

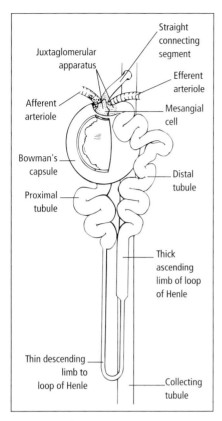

Figure 3.15 A nephron.

Renal tubules

Proximal tubule

About 75% of the excess water is reabsorbed in the proximal tubule, which is lined with active cells whose surface area is enormously increased by their *brush border* of microvilli (Fig. 3.17). These metabolically busy cells also recover glucose, phosphate and amino acids from the glomerular filtrate.

Loop of Henle

The filtrate now passes through the *loops of Henle*. Most of these are quite short, but those in the inner part of the pyramid dip down like hairpins into the papilla, where they run alongside collecting tubules. The cells of the loops of Henle are thin, and allow osmosis to withdraw salt and water from the glomerular filtrate into the concentrated tissue of the papilla. So-called 'loop diuretics', e.g. frusemide, inhibit Cl^- transport, reduce hypertonicity in the papilla, and allow more water to escape along with potassium. This effect is further potentiated by spironolactone.

Tests of glomerular filtration

For most purposes the plasma *creatinine* is an adequate guide to glomerular function. Occasionally a more precise measure is needed. The classical test used to be the *creatinine clearance*. This required an exactly timed collection of urine, which was difficult in a busy hospital ward. The plasma creatinine was then measured at some convenient time. Clearance was given by the formula UV/P, where U is the urine creatinine mg/100 mL, V is the urine volume in mL/min and P is the plasma creatinine mg/100 mL. The answer was expressed in mL/min. The exactly timed collection of urine was a source of error and for this reason creatinine clearance has been superseded by diethylene triamine pentacetic acid (DTPA) clearance. ^{99m}Tc-labelled DTPA is given and the rate of disappearance from the kidney or forearm measured with a gamma camera.

Distal tubule

The filtrate now rises up into the distal convoluted tubule whose cells are thick and metabolically active but have no brush border. They exchange Na for K and H ions to regulate the acid–base balance of the body. Disease of the distal convoluted tubules prevents the urine from forming an acid urine, the so-called renal tubular acidosis.

Collecting tubules

Leaving the distal convoluted tubule the filtrate enters the collecting tubule, and once more runs the gauntlet of the hypertonic papilla. Here the last fine-tuning of the reabsorption of water takes place under the control of the pituitary antidiuretic hormone.

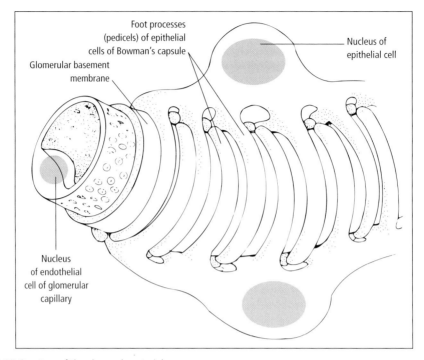

Foot processes
(pedicels) of epithelial
cells of Bowman's capsule

Glomerular basement
membrane

Nucleus of
epithelial cell

Nucleus
of endothelial
cell of glomerular
capillary

Figure 3.16 Structure of the glomerular arteriole.

Tests of tubular function

DMSA

The rate of uptake of ^{99m}Tc DMSA is recorded by a gamma camera. This is the usual test of renal tubular function. Only occasionally is it necessary to use the classical tests.

Acid load

After collecting two 1-hour specimens of urine over 2 hours, the patient is given NH_4Cl in gelatin-coated capsules (0.1 g/kg body weight) in a litre of water over 1 hour. Three hours later a third 1-hour specimen of urine is collected. Healthy distal tubules can handle this by secreting urine with a pH over 5.3, a titratable acidity over 25 mmol/min and over 35 mmol/min of ammonium. In practice, the NH_4Cl often makes patients vomit and the test is void.

Urine concentration test

The patient may be deprived of water, or given desmopressin, an analogue of pituitary antidiuretic hormone (40 μg/kg for adults, 20 μg/kg for children) and the specific gravity of the urine is measured over the next 6 hours. The test must never be attempted in patients with renal failure.

Blood supply of the kidney

Renal arteries

Between them the kidneys receive one-fifth of the entire cardiac output. Usually there is one renal artery on each side, with five segmental branches arranged like the digits of the hand (Fig. 3.18).

• Each segmental branch supplies its own geographical zone of the parenchyma. They are *end-arteries* and there are no anastomoses between them (Fig. 3.19). The zones supplied by the *segmental arteries* do not match the arrangement of

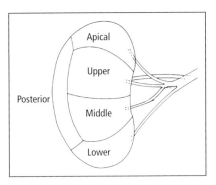

Figure 3.19 Each segmental artery supplies its own geographical territory.

cortex and medulla, giving off branches which run up and down parallel with the collecting tubules, as well as giving an *afferent artery* to each glomerulus (Fig. 3.20).

• The afferent artery enters the glomerulus near the junction of the loop of Henle with the distal convoluted tubule: the *juxtaglomerular apparatus* is located here; its cells contain dark granules of the precursor of renin. The juxtaglomerular apparatus monitors the pressure in the afferent arteriole.

Renal veins

Unlike the segmental branches of the renal arteries, the veins communicate freely with each other (Fig. 3.21). Several veins can be ligated without infarcting the kidney. The main left renal vein often splits into two, one part running in front of the aorta, the other behind, posing a trap for the surgeon who is unaware of this anomaly. The left renal vein is about 5 cm long; the right is close to the inferior vena cava, another reason why the left kidney is preferred in live donor transplantation.

The collecting system

The thin cubical epithelium of the papilla is perforated with the collecting ducts (of *Bellini*) but the rest of the pelvis and calix is lined by urothelium like that of the bladder and ureters. The urothelium is surrounded by a wall of smooth muscle cells linked by jigsaw connections, *nexuses*, which

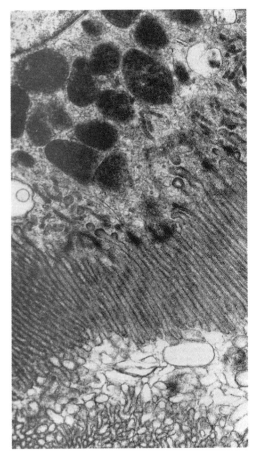

Figure 3.17 Electron photomicrograph showing the brush border of the proximal renal tubule.

pyramids and calices. In open operations any incision into the renal parenchyma is made between the main segmental arteries, which can be located with a Doppler probe.

• Each segmental artery divides into smaller *arcuate arteries* which run in the boundary between

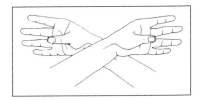

Figure 3.18 Arrangement of the branches of the renal arteries.

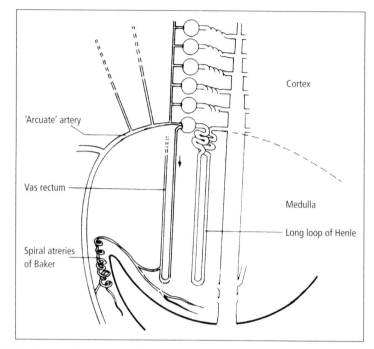

Figure 3.20 The blood supply of the renal papilla.

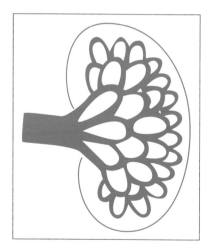

Figure 3.21 The veins of the kidney communicate with each other.

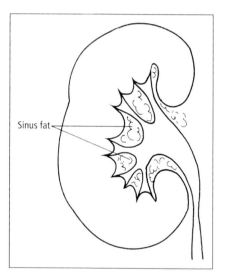

Figure 3.22 The calices are surrounded by sinus fat which is fluid at body temperature and allows them to move freely.

transmit the wave of contraction from one muscle cell to another without the need for any nerve supply, so a transplanted kidney continues to pump out urine perfectly well.

The calices are separated from the renal parenchyma by a packing of sinus fat which is fluid at body temperature, and allows them to contract freely (Fig. 3.22).

Chapter 4

The kidney: congenital disorders

Embryology

Primitive vertebrates were constructed like a railway train: each identical somite had a pair of nephrons which allowed fluid from the coelom to leak out into the surrounding sea. Later on these nephrons came to be arranged into three groups:
• The most cranial of these, the *pronephros*, is today only an evolutionary curiosity, found in a few fish embryos, but of no relevance to humans.
• The second set, the *mesonephros*, corresponds to the kidney of present day fish and frogs whose mesonephric (Wolffian) duct empties urine into the cloaca.
• Human kidneys are derived from a third, most caudal set of nephrons – the *metanephros* – which drains into the ureter (Fig. 4.1).

Mesonephric (Wolffian) ducts

In humans the mesonephros has disappeared, but its duct persists as the *vas deference* in males and the caudal part of the ureter.

If the mesonephric duct fails to develop then there will be neither ureter, kidney nor a vas deferens on that side – renal agenesis (Fig. 4.2).

Lecture Notes: Urology, 6th edition. By John Blandy and Amir Kaisary. Published 2009 by Blackwell Publishing. ISBN: 978-1-4051-2270-2.

Paramesonephric (Müllerian) ducts

These are a second pair of ducts parallel with the mesonephric ducts:
• In females, they form the *Fallopian tubes*, which fuse in the midline to form the *uterus*.
• In males, they persist as a pit on the verumontanum in the prostatic urethra – the *utriculus masculinus* – as well as a tiny cyst attached to the upper pole of the testis which sometimes twists on its stalk and mimics torsion of the testicle.

The urogenital septum

While the ureters are growing up towards the metanephros (Fig. 4.3) a shutter of tissue, the *urogenital septum*, grows down to separate the bladder from the rectum, carrying with it the mesonephric duct and the ureteric buds which are bent into a loop.
• The lower part of the mesonephric duct is absorbed into the *trigone* of the future bladder (Fig. 4.4).
• In males the upper part of the mesonephric duct – taken over as the vas deferens – swings down with the testis into the scrotum (Fig. 4.5).

Duplex kidney and ureter

After budding out from the lower end of the mesonephric duct, the ureter usually begins to

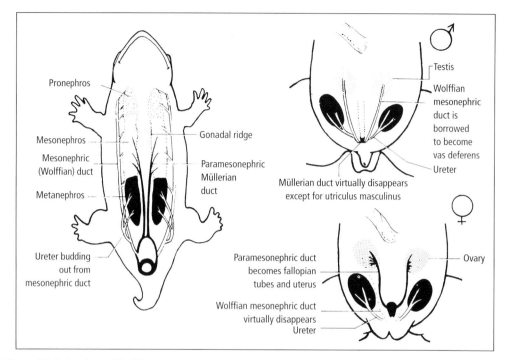

Figure 4.1 Embryology of the kidney.

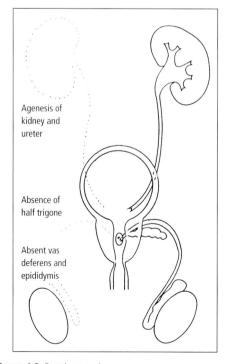

Figure 4.2 Renal agenesis.

branch when it gets near the metanephros but sometimes it divides earlier and may produce a complete double system of renal pelvis and calyces – *ren duplex*. The overlying renal parenchyma is never completely separated but a distinct 'waist' marks the distinction between the two halves, as does a prominent bulge in the parenchyma, which may be mistaken for a carcinoma in X-rays (Fig. 4.6).

• The upper half of the kidney has two main calyces, the lower half has three and makes more urine.

• Urine may be squirted from the lower half up into the upper half, causing distension and pain – yo-yo reflux (Fig. 4.7).

A duplex kidney is nearly always innocent and symptomless, but it can be associated with three conditions that cause trouble:

• *Ectopic ureter:* The ureter draining the upper half of the kidney may open into the vagina, caudal to the sphincter, and gives rise to continual incontinence (Fig. 4.8).

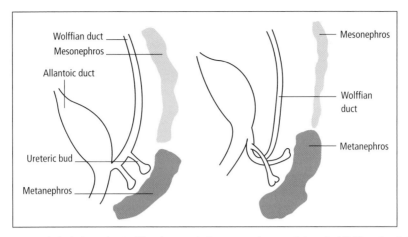

Figure 4.3 Two ureteric buds from the Wolffian duct reach the metanephros, and then the Wolffian duct is bent round.

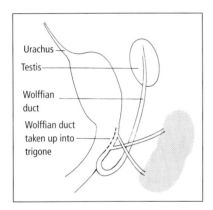

Figure 4.4 The lower end of the Wolffian duct is incorporated into the bladder.

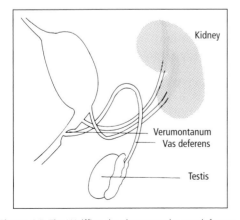

Figure 4.5 The Wolffian duct becomes the vas deferens.

- *Reflux:* The ureter from the lower half of the kidney has a short course through the wall of the bladder thus less efficient as a valve, and urine may reflux from the bladder up to the kidney (Fig. 4.9).
- *Ureterocele:* If the lower end of the mesonephric duct is incompletely absorbed into the trigone, it may form a balloon just where the ureter enters the trigone – *ureterocele*. This is most often seen at the lower of two ureteric orifices in duplex. Very occasionally a ureterocele may prolapse out of the urethra as a translucent 'cyst' causing painful acute retention of urine (Fig. 4.10).

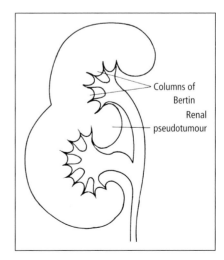

Figure 4.6 In duplex kidney there is often a very prominent column of Bertin.

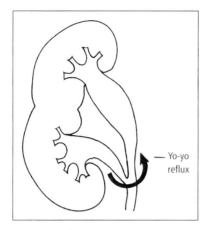

Figure 4.7 Yo-yo reflux.

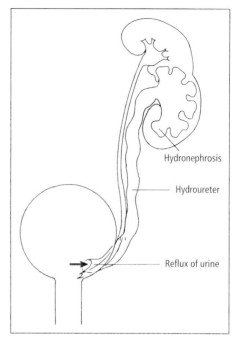

Figure 4.9 Reflux up the upper ureteric orifice into the lower half of the kidney.

Errors of position of the kidney

Rotated kidney

A kidney often faces forwards rather than medially. Its outline is then an ellipse and some of its calices point medially (Fig. 4.11). This condition is harmless.

Horseshoe kidney

If both the metanephroi get fused together in the foetal pelvis, not only are both kidneys rotated, but also their lower poles are joined in the shape of a horseshoe (Fig. 4.12). The cause for this is unknown. As the foetus grows, the joined kidneys are held up by the inferior or superior mesenteric arteries. In operations for aortic aneurysm, the isthmus joining the two kidneys may have to be divided, but otherwise it should be left alone.

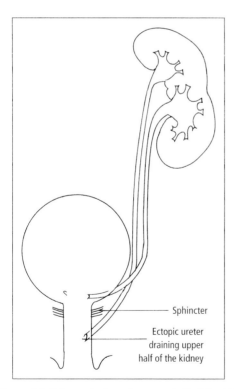

Figure 4.8 If the ureter from the upper half of the kidney opens below the sphincter in a girl there is continual incontinence.

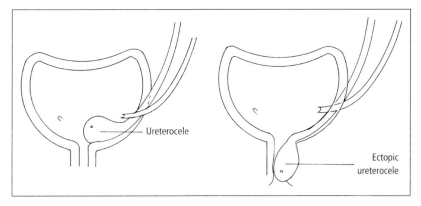

Figure 4.10 A ureterocele may prolapse into the urethra.

This condition is often associated with reflux, ureterocele and hydronephrosis.

Each of these conditions should be dealt with in the usual way, without meddling with the isthmus.

Crossed renal ectopia

Instead of being united in the midline like a horseshoe, the two kidneys may fuse together on one side. Their ureters always run along their proper side. As with horseshoe kidney, there is often some other congenital anomaly such as reflux or obstruction (Fig. 4.13).

Pelvic kidney

Here the metanephros remains in the pelvis. One might expect it would get in the way of the baby during childbirth, but it hardly ever does. A pelvic kidney is usually detected by chance, and seldom needs any treatment unless associated with some other condition such as hydronephrosis. But there is one unexpected and important hazard: at laparotomy for abdominal pain an unwary surgeon may come across an unusual 'tumour' and go ahead to remove it. In pelvic kidneys the segmental arteries arise directly from the aorta, common and internal iliac arteries. If the condition is not recognised there can by confusion and bleeding (Fig. 4.14).

Thoracic kidney

This is not so much an error of development of the kidney as of the diaphragm, where one kidney is carried up into the chest along with other viscera. Such a 'thoracic' kidney is found by chance in a chest radiograph or an intravenous urogram (IVU).

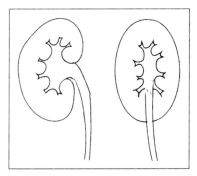

Figure 4.11 Rotated kidney.

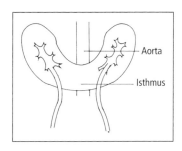

Figure 4.12 Horseshoe kidney.

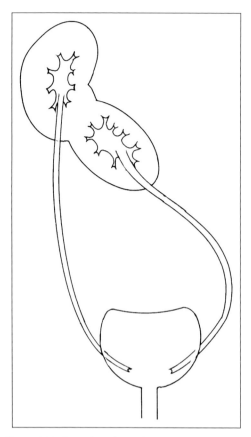

Figure 4.13 Crossed renal ectopia.

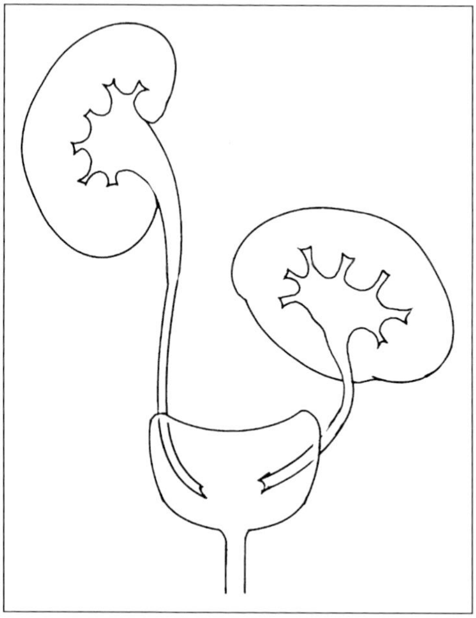

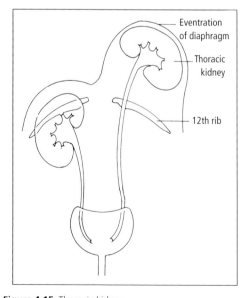

Figure 4.14 Pelvic kidney.

The kidney is not really in the thorax: a thin layer of diaphragm and pleura always separates the two compartments. The kidney itself needs no treatment (Fig. 4.15).

Errors of development of the kidney

Agenesis

If the mesonephric duct fails to develop there is an absence of ureter, trigone, kidney and (in boys) vas deferens (see Fig. 4.2).

Aplasia

The metanephros may not differentiate at all – aplasia (Fig. 4.16).

Figure 4.15 Thoracic kidney.

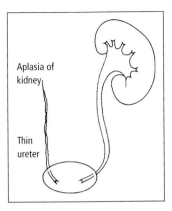

Figure 4.16 Aplasia.

Dysplasia

The metanephros may develop poorly, with odd-looking tissue including little cysts and lumps of cartilage (Fig. 4.17).

Hypoplasia

This is a term to avoid: it implies that the kidney is small but otherwise normal. This is never the case: it is either dysplastic or scarred, or both.

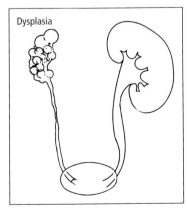

Figure 4.17 Dysplasia.

Cystic disorders of the kidney

Medullary sponge kidney

Here the collecting ducts are grossly dilated (Fig. 4.18). Part or all of one or both kidneys may be affected, and the medulla becomes honeycombed with cysts giving the appearance of a sponge. The radiographic appearance is characteristic (Fig. 4.19).

Infection in the dilated tubules is soon followed by the development of numerous small *stones* which give repeated attacks of ureteric colic. With extracorporeal lithotripsy the larger stones can be broken up and allowed to pass before they give rise to serious trouble, but repeated attacks of infection and scarring ultimately lead to renal failure.

Obstruction cysts

Congenital obstruction of the ureter

The ureter may become narrowed in foetal life for causes as yet unknown.

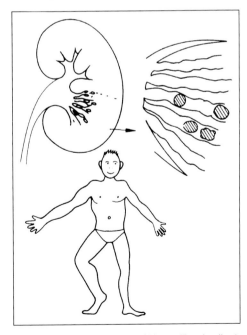

Figure 4.18 Medullary sponge kidney: dilated collecting tubules and unilateral hemihypertrophy of the body.

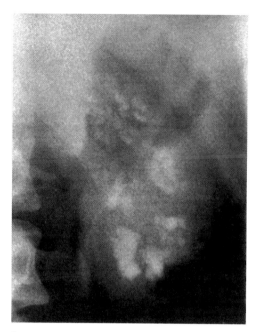

Figure 4.19 X-ray of medullary sponge kidney showing multiple calculi in dilated collecting ducts.

• The kidney continues to make urine, and the nephrons become distended, converting the kidney into a so-called *congenital multicystic kidney* (Fig. 4.20). If the condition is bilateral the foetus forms no urine, so there is no amniotic fluid, and the baby's face is characteristically flattened – *Potter's facies* (Fig. 4.21). There are usually other

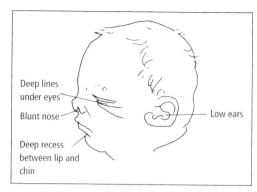

Figure 4.21 Potter's facies.

congenital anomalies and the condition is incompatible with life.

• A minor version of this imperfect development of the ureter is seen where there is a tiny, thin ureter, above which a small kidney is found, largely converted into small cysts – cystic dysplasia.

• A single calix may become obstructed, and the pyramid draining into it becomes converted into a hollow bag – *caliceal cyst*. These are found when infection or stones develop in the cyst (Fig. 4.22).

Acquired obstruction

Scarring

Rather similar cysts occur as a consequence of the scarring and contraction which takes place in the later stages of *pyelonephritis*. The obstructed nephrons occasionally become grossly distended with protein (Fig. 4.23). This kind of cyst is often seen in patients who survive for many years with end-stage renal failure on dialysis.

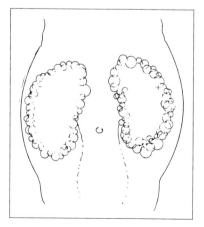

Figure 4.20 Congenital multicystic kidney.

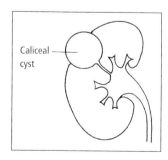

Caliceal cyst

Figure 4.22 Caliceal cyst.

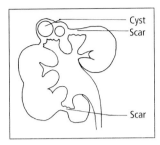

Figure 4.23 Obstructed cysts in pyelonephritic scarring.

Diverticula of the collecting tubules

The most common type of *simple renal cyst* arises as a *diverticulum* from the collecting tubules of the kidney. Simple cysts occur in middle age in almost every normal kidney and are detected by accident in an ultrasound scan (Fig. 4.24). Usually nothing needs to be done about them (Fig. 4.25). Occasionally these simple cysts may grow big enough to obstruct a calyx and cause pain, especially if they arise from the medulla (*parapelvic cysts*). They can be emptied by fine-needle aspiration, and if they fill up again, can be uncapped at an open or percutaneous procedure. Very rarely the fluid inside a cyst becomes infected and requires drainage.

Polycystic disease

A bizarre exaggeration of this process is seen in polycystic disease. There are two main forms of this condition: childhood and adult.

(a) **Childhood polycystic disease** (Fig. 4.26). This type of polycystic disease is inherited as a

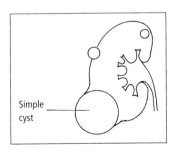

Figure 4.24 Simple cysts of the kidney.

Mendelian recessive characteristic and is picked up at four different ages.

1 *Foetal:* Ultrasound in pregnancy reveals that both kidneys have been converted into giant sponges. It is not compatible with survival.

2 *Neonatal:* A similar condition is discovered in the neonate, who may survive for up to a year, unless a transplant can be found.

3 *Infantile:* Between 3 and 6 months, these children are found to have uraemia and enlarged kidneys; there is also an associated fibrosis of the portal system.

4 *Juvenile:* This is discovered in later childhood, and is also associated with hepatic fibrosis.

(b) **Adult polycystic disease** (Fig. 4.27). This is inherited by an autosomal dominant gene on chromosome 16. It may appear in children, but is usually diagnosed in adult life. It may be associated with cysts in the liver and pancreas and berry aneurysms of the circle of Willis which cause subarachnoid haemorrhage. Many patients have no symptoms at all. Often the diagnosis is made by accident when an abdominal lump is found on routine palpation or ultrasound scanning.

Complications include the following:

1 *Hypertension:* This can be treated medically for many years.

2 *Uraemia:* At first this can be managed with restriction of protein. Later the patient may need dialysis, and ultimately may require a transplant.

3 *Infection:* It is rare for these cysts to become infected, but occasionally they do, and call for drainage. There is no other indication to drain these cysts. (The so-called Rövsing operation has been shown to do more harm than good.)

Congenital disorders of the renal tubules

Proximal tubules

A number of congenital errors involve the enzymes which transport amino acids across the mucosa of the bowel and the epithelium of the proximal renal tubule. The most important are as follows.

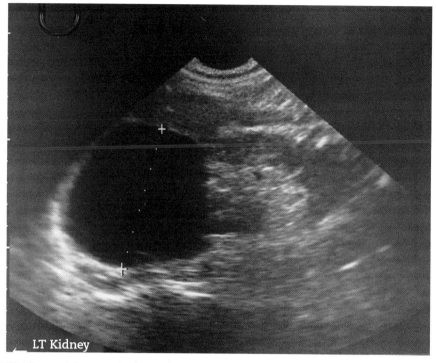

Figure 4.25 Ultrasound showing a simple cyst. (Courtesy of Dr W. Hately.)

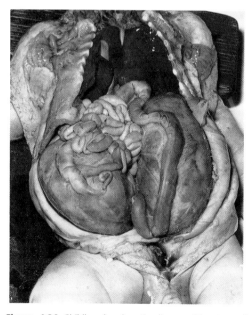

Figure 4.26 Childhood polycystic disease. (Courtesy of the late Mr J. H. Johnston.)

Cystinuria

Four amino acids are affected: cystine, ornithine, arginine and lysine ('coal') of which the only important one is *cystine* because it is poorly soluble in urine. The deficiency is inherited as a Mendelian autosomal recessive: only 3% of patients are homozygous. Heterozygous patients lose about 500 mg/24 hours of cystine in their urine: homozygous patients lose twice as much and so their urine is bound to be supersaturated for cystine. Cystine stones are radiodense because of their sulphur content. Penicillamine binds the cystine in a soluble form and if combined with a high fluid input may prevent stones from forming and even dissolve those that are present (Fig. 4.28).

Hartnup disease

Here tryptophane cannot be absorbed from the bowel resulting in nicotinamide deficiency, pellagra and cerebellar ataxia.

Renal glycosuria

Here the tubules fail to reabsorb glucose which appears in the urine even when the blood sugar is normal. It is quite harmless but has to be distinguished from diabetes mellitus.

Phosphate

If the tubules fail to reabsorb phosphate from the glomerular filtrate the result is *vitamin D-resistant rickets*.

Distal renal tubules

Renal tubular acidosis

Disease of the distal tubule may make it unable to pump out hydrogen ions so that the kidney cannot form acidic urine and loses potassium, phosphate, sulphate and other organic acids. The resulting low plasma bicarbonate increases the proportion of calcium that is not bound to a protein particle, so more calcium escapes in the filtrate where it is precipitated in the tubules, leading to speckled calcification – *nephrocalcinosis*. At first, these patients have normal glomerular function, but the continual loss of calcium and phosphate leads to *osteomalacia*. The diagnosis is made by the acid load test and the remedy is potassium bicarbonate or citrate and additional vitamin D.

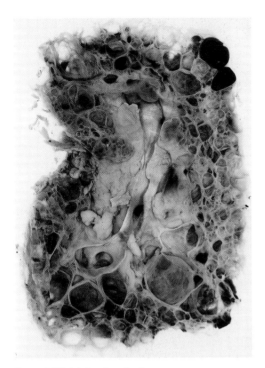

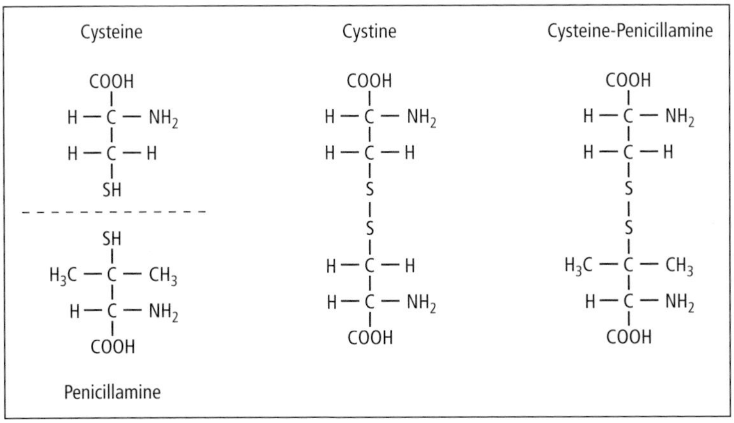

Figure 4.27 Adult polycystic disease.

Fanconi's syndrome

A disorder where there is malabsorption of several amino acids as well as phosphate. This is accompanied by proteinuria and acidosis as well.

Figure 4.28 Cystine, cysteine and penicillamine.

Collecting tubules

A sex-linked Mendelian recessive gene in males may prevent collecting tubules from responding to the pituitary antidiuretic hormone – *nephrogenic diabetes insipidus*. Continued diuresis may lead to dehydration, severe enough to cause brain damage in the baby and gross dilatation of the kidneys and ureters.

Acquired disorders of the renal tubules

Obstructive uropathy

Back-pressure atrophy of the renal papillae is often seen in chronic obstruction. Glomerular filtration may be more or less unaffected, but the kidney is no longer able to acidify or concentrate the urine. The urine from the obstructed side is pale and has a fixed specific gravity. When both kidneys have been obstructed for a long time the patient may become severely dehydrated.

Sickle-cell disease

In the sickle-cell trait, even though there may never be a crisis, small vessels in the renal papilla may become blocked by the malformed red cells. The result is a series of ischaemic changes which result in an inability of the tubules to concentrate or acidify the urine. Microscopic haematuria is nearly always present.

Chapter 5

The kidney: trauma

Penetrating injuries

The kidney may be injured by a knife or bullet wound. In knife injuries, and those caused by low-velocity bullets, the kidney can usually be repaired. In high-velocity missile injuries the blast devitalises a large sphere of tissue, and if the kidney is within this sphere, it must be removed or else there is likely to be fatal secondary haemorrhage.

Closed injuries

Closed injuries of the kidney are often seen in sport. To damage the kidney the blow has to be quite severe and so it often fractures the lower ribs and tips of the transverse processes of the lumbar vertebrae (Fig. 5.1).

There are three grades of closed renal injury (Fig. 5.2):

1 The parenchyma is *split*, causing haematuria and a haematoma is confined by the strong thin bag of Gerota's fascia. The bleeding soon stops and the parenchyma heals completely within a few weeks.

2 The kidney splits into several *fragments*. Again Gerota's fascia limits the expansion of the

Lecture Notes: Urology, 6th edition. By John Blandy and Amir Kaisary. Published 2009 by Blackwell Publishing. ISBN: 978-1-4051-2270-2.

haematoma. The bleeding usually stops spontaneously and the kidney is expected to heal without any obvious sequel.

3 There is, in addition, a tear of the main *renal artery* or *vein* causing massive bleeding.

History

There is a story of an injury to the loin followed by haematuria.

Management

On admission the patient is carefully examined to rule out pneumothorax, and internal bleeding into the chest or peritoneal cavity from associated injury to the liver or spleen. Every patient is admitted for observation because there is no way of telling how severe the original laceration of the kidney is, or how it is going to progress during the next few hours.

Investigations

The chest is X-rayed. An emergency intravenous urogram (IVU) is performed not so much to show the type of the injury, but to make sure there is a kidney on the other side. Recently, it has become more common to perform computed tomography (CT) in the early investigation of such patients. This can cause some confusion because the

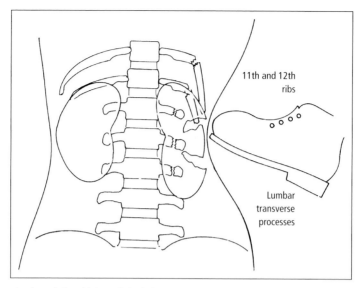

11th and 12th ribs

Lumbar transverse processes

Figure 5.1 The mechanism of closed injury of the kidney.

appearance of the ruptured kidney in the CT scan can be frightening. It is not an indication for open surgery. If the CT scan is performed after the patient has started to deteriorate it may cause dangerous delay. The patient is then kept under close observation, the pulse, blood pressure and abdominal girth being recorded at regular intervals. Every specimen of urine is saved for inspection. Nearly all these patients get steadily better. The colour of the blood in successive specimens of urine becomes less and less bright and the patient remains well. But one cannot predict that this will happen all the time. Every so often, things go wrong: there is a rising pulse, falling blood pressure and abdominal distension suggesting internal bleeding.

When there is clinical deterioration the most useful investigation at this stage is a renal angiogram. This may identify the artery which is bleeding, and allow it to be plugged with gelfoam or chopped muscle injected through the catheter (Fig. 5.3). If this is not possible, or if the patient is obviously deteriorating, laparotomy must not be delayed. The kidney is approached through a midline incision. The surgeon first secures the aorta and renal vessels before opening Gerota's fascia,

which, until then, will have been limiting the bleeding by tamponade. Once the renal artery is secured and the clot evacuated, it may be possible to repair the damage. More often a nephrectomy is needed.

Follow-up

Five important complications must be borne in mind:

1 *Secondary haemorrhage:* When there has been a severe laceration the clot that is holding the pieces of kidney together may undergo lysis. Late secondary haemorrhage may occur at any time within the first 2 weeks, but is exceedingly rare when the initial tear in the kidney was only a small one (Fig. 5.4).

2 *Renal artery stenosis:* A small laceration of the renal artery may heal with stenosis and cause hypertension (Fig. 5.5).

3 *Page kidney:* An organising haematoma may form a thick tough shell around the kidney which then shrinks, compressing the kidney leading to ischaemia and hypertension (Fig. 5.6).

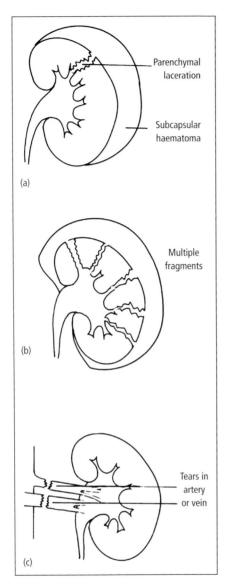

(a)

Parenchymal laceration

Subcapsular haematoma

(b)

Multiple fragments

(c)

Tears in artery or vein

Figure 5.2 Three grades of renal injury.

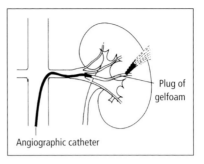

Plug of gelfoam

Angiographic catheter

Figure 5.3 Bleeding from a segmental artery can be blocked by injection of gelfoam through an angiography catheter.

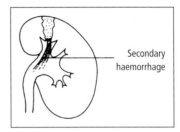

Secondary haemorrhage

Figure 5.4 Secondary haemorrhage.

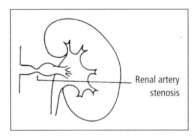

Renal artery stenosis

Figure 5.5 Renal artery stenosis.

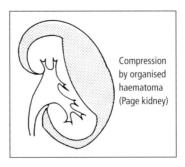

Compression by organised haematoma (Page kidney)

Figure 5.6 Page kidney.

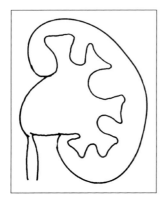

Figure 5.7 Hydronephrosis.

4 *Hydronephrosis:* It is rare to have evidence that a kidney was formerly normal, and only became hydronephrotic after injury. It is common for a hydronephrosis to be discovered after an injury. Just as distended balloon is more likely to burst than a floppy one, a distended hydronephrosis is more prone to trauma. Seldom is it possible to be sure which came first: the hydronephrosis or the injury (Fig. 5.7).

5 *Pseudocyst or urinoma:* This is a rare but potentially lethal complication. If the split in the renal pelvis allows urine to escape into the surround-

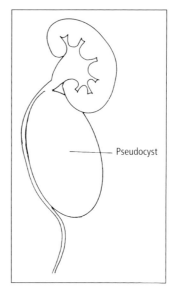

Figure 5.8 Pseudocyst or urinoma.

ing tissue it may form a large collection – a urinoma (Fig. 5.8) – which becomes surrounded by a fibrous tissue wall which sometimes calcifies. Sooner or later the collection of urine becomes infected and needs to be drained. It may require total excision.

Chapter 6

The kidney: inflammation

Immunological disorders

Anything can act as an antigen either by itself or in combination with various peptides. The long list of antigens that can cause allergic inflammation in the kidney ranges from simple chemicals such as penicillamine and butazolidine, to entire microorganisms such as *Streptococcus* and *Plasmodium malariae*. Even the patient's own DNA can sometimes act as the allergen. The immune system of a healthy patient reacts to an unwanted antigen by smothering it with *insoluble complex*, which is scavenged by the reticuloendothelial system before it can reach the kidney. If there is too little antibody to smother the antigen completely, smaller *soluble complexes* may form which get trapped in the stalk of the glomerulus – (the mesangium) or between the slit pores of the basement membrane.

Nephrotic syndrome

Soluble complexes usually cause little damage. A renal biopsy shows nothing wrong on light microscopy and even the electron microscope shows only minimal damage to the basement membrane (Fig. 6.1). The diagnosis of nephrotic syndrome is made by the presence of the findings listed below:

proteinuria (more than 3.5 g a day);
hypoalbuminaemia;
oedema; and
hypercholesterolaemia.

Main aetiological factors involved in the development of nephrotic syndrome include glomerulonephritis, drug reactions and allergic reactions. Drug-induced nephropathy may be caused by drugs such as penicillamine or even consumption of heavy metals such as gold, mercury and cadmium. Allergic reactions to allergens such as beestings, pollen or even lactose in cow's milk, may cause the nephrotic syndrome.

Although there are many subtypes of nephrotic syndrome, the main cause of nephrotic syndrome is caused by membranous glomerulonephritis in approximately 25% of cases, closely followed by minimal change nephropathy (or lipoid nephropathy) in 20% of cases.

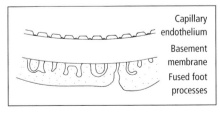

Figure 6.1 Minimal change disease of the basement membrane.

Lecture Notes: Urology, 6th edition. By John Blandy and Amir Kaisary. Published 2009 by Blackwell Publishing. ISBN: 978-1-4051-2270-2.

Clinical picture

Clinically the picture is one of gross *oedema*. The *nephrotic syndrome* is usually seen in children. Most patients with nephrotic syndrome recover spontaneously. However, the recovery of these patients is aided with dietary sodium restriction. Use of thiazide diuretics (e.g. bendrofluazide) may help reduce fluid accumulation. A normal protein diet is usually adequate as a high-protein diet usually confers no additional benefits.

Nephritic syndrome

Nephritic syndrome development can be attributed to humoral mechanisms leading to the deposition of antibodies within the glomerulus. These antibodies form immune complexes that set off the cascade of inflammation, which results in the perforation of cell membranes, the release of histamine from mast cells and platelets, dilatation of blood vessels and an influx of leucocytes. If the leucocytes remain within the mesangium or glomerular tuft the changes are usually reversible (Fig. 6.2), but if they burst out into the space of Bowman's capsule it becomes choked with cells and the outlook is far worse (Fig. 6.3).

Diagnosis of acute nephritic syndrome can be made by the presence of:

haematuria (microscopic or macroscopic);
proteinuria;
hypertension;

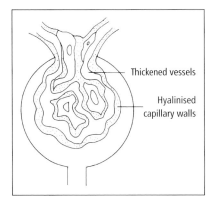

Figure 6.2 Mesangiocapillary disease: inflammatory exudate in the mesangium and the glomerular tuft.

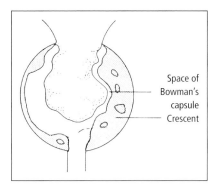

Figure 6.3 Extracapillary proliferative disease: exudate fills up Bowman's capsule.

oliguria;
uraemia; and
oedema (usually lower limb, periorbital or sacral oedema).

The causes of acute nephritic syndrome can be classified according to whether it is of immunological origin or otherwise. Clear immunological causes of the nephritic syndrome are conditions such as: (1) post-streptococcal glomerulonephritis (usually attributed to Lancefield group A β-haemolytic streptococci); (2) IgA nephropathy; (3) membranous nephropathy (e.g. secondary to SLE, gold and penicillamine); (4) Henoch-Schönlein purpura; and (5) anti-glomerular basement membrane disease. The aetiology of conditions such as minimal change nephropathy, focal glomerulosclerosis, haemolytic–uraemic syndrome and Wegener's granulomatosis, do not have clearly established immunological mechanisms.

Clinical picture

The clinical picture of the nephritic syndrome is more dramatic. There is a rapid onset with *haematuria*, *hypertension* and (if the tubules are clogged with red and white cells) there may be *anuria*. If the kidneys fail to clear themselves, they heal with scarring. The clinical management in these patients is mainly conservative and involves managing the hypertension and generalised body oedema. Dietary protein restriction may be required in severe uraemia; however, fluid and sodium restriction is always necessary.

Matrix deposit diseases

There are three main disorders in which matrix are deposited throughout the kidney:
• *Diabetic nephropathy*: An eosinophilic matrix is deposited in the glomerular arteriolr, causing its wall to thicken. There is loss of albumen and red cells, and hypertension follows.
• *Amyloidosis*: Amyloid is deposited in the glomerulus to give a glassy eosinophilic deposit throughout the glomerulus and Bowman's capsule. The whole picture may be suddenly worsened by thrombosis of the renal vein.
• *Myelomatosis*: In multiple myeloma the bone marrow produces an excess of immunoglobulins. Light-chain immunoglobulins may appear in the urine as the *Bence-Jones protein* which coagulates when the urine is warmed to 50°C and dissolves again as it is warmed up even further.

Urinary tract infection

Uncomplicated lower urinary tract infection

This condition refers to a urinary tract infection that is confined to the urinary bladder and is more common in females compared with males. The shorter length of the female urethra predisposes to the introduction of pathogenic organisms into the bladder from the distal urethra and perineum. As many as one third of women in their thirties would have had at least one episode of lower urinary tract infection. Common bacterial organisms that cause lower urinary tract infections include *Escherichia coli, Klebsiella, Streptococcus faecalis* or *Proteus mirabilis*.

Upper urinary tract infection/pyelonephritis

Presence of lower urinary tract infections can cause upper urinary tract infections (or pyelonephritis), which involves the kidneys. Ureters that permit vesicoureteric reflux of infected urine into the kidneys may cause pyelonephritis. Other factors that predispose to upper urinary tract infections in-clude poor ureteric peristalsis, ureteric obstruction, renal scarring and poor renal blood flow.

Haematogenous infection

Blood-borne infection may also carry microorganisms to the kidney where they form multiple small abscesses in the renal parenchyma. These are normally dealt with by the usual defence mechanisms and heal without significant scarring. They are often seen postmortem in patients who have had a terminal episode of bacteraemia. A previous scar in the kidney makes it more susceptible to such haematogenous infection. Important blood-borne infections include those due to staphylococci and *Mycobacterium tuberculosis*.

Factors predisposing to urinary infection (Fig. 6.4)

Some factors that predispose to urinary tract infections include the following.

Urinary stasis
Urine is an excellent culture medium in which microorganisms multiply at body temperature unless the pool of urine is regularly and completely

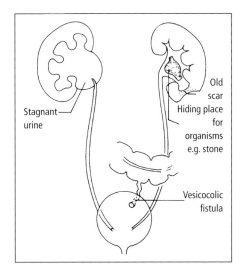

Figure 6.4 Factors contributing to urinary infection.

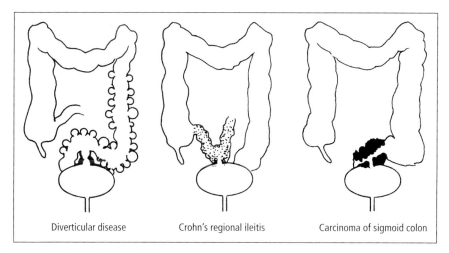

Diverticular disease Crohn's regional ileitis Carcinoma of sigmoid colon

Figure 6.5 Infection from enterovesical fistulae.

emptied out. Stagnant pools of urine occur during the following circumstances:

• *Infrequent voiding:* Some people empty their bladders very infrequently. As bacteria divide every 15 minutes, an inoculum of only 10 bacteria may in theory increase to 8×10^6 within 6 hours. A practical way to prevent urinary infection is for patients to undergo bladder re-training, where they are persuaded to empty their bladders every hour.

• *Obstruction:* Whatever the cause, e.g. hydronephrosis, a stone or an obstructing prostate gland, the end result is the same – a pool of stagnant urine which sooner or later becomes infected.

• *Undrained pockets of urine:* Diverticula occur anywhere in the urinary tract, especially in the bladder and kidney, forming a pool of urine that never empties out completely.

• *Dilated and refluxing ureters:* Many conditions cause the ureters to become dilated. There may be obstruction, e.g. by a stone or a tumour, or the ureterovesical valve may be deficient. The end result is the same – a pool of urine that is never completely drained out, and invites infection.

Hiding places for microorganisms

• *Stones:* Stones are often crumbly, and a biofilm between the crystals allows organisms to lurk, sheltered from antibiotics that cannot diffuse into the centre of the stone.

• *Necrotic tissue:* Very similar hiding places for bacteria are provided by necrotic tissue, e.g. necrotic tissue in a cancer, or a foreign body such as a nylon stitch or a fragment of a catheter.

Sources of reinfection

Microorganisms may be repeatedly injected into the urinary tract from a fistula into adjacent bowel, e.g.

• diverticular disease of the colon;
• cancer of the colon; and
• Crohn's disease of the small bowel (Fig. 6.5).

Lowered resistance to infection

It is a clinical commonplace to note that the symptoms of an ordinary urinary infection often begin a few days after an influenza-like illness which has impaired host resistance. More significant and important causes of impaired host resistance are:

• diabetes mellitus;
• acquired immune deficiency syndrome (AIDS); and
• immunosuppression for transplantation or during cancer chemotherapy.

End result of urinary infection

Infection in the kidney, like infection anywhere else in the body, can be followed by one of four processes (Fig. 6.6):

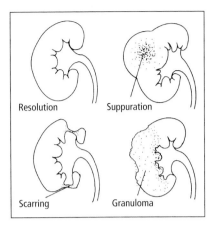

Figure 6.6 Four possible outcomes from renal infection.

- *Resolution:* This is the usual result. Most patients with bacterial infection in the bladder or kidney end up with an absolutely normal bladder and an undamaged kidney.
- *Suppuration:* When the kidney is obstructed the entire kidney may be converted into a bag of pus – *pyonephrosis.* A minor form of this is seen when one calix is obstructed – *pyocalix.* Suppuration after haematogenous infection may cause an abscess in the renal cortex which spreads into the surrounding fat to cause a *renal carbuncle* (see p. 59).
- *Scarring:* Scarring occurs when there has been both obstruction and infection: it may be diffuse – *interstitial nephritis* – or localised, to produce a deeply pitted *scar in the parenchyma* (see reflux nephropathy below).
- *Granuloma:* Organisms which cause chronic inflammation elsewhere, e.g. tuberculosis, brucellosis and actinomycosis, can cause granuloma formation in the kidney. There are also a group of very unusual granulomas which follow infection with *E. coli.*

Reflux nephropathy

Many children are born with defective valves at the entry of the ureters into the bladder, especially when there are other congenital anomalies such as duplex kidney or ureterocele. When the bladder contracts the urine is forced back up to the ureter to the kidney. If in addition, the *compound papillae*

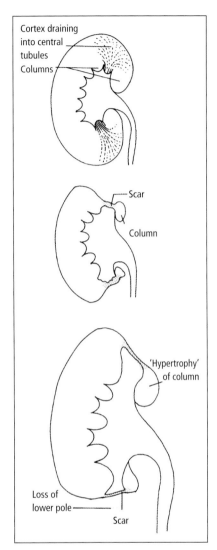

Figure 6.7 Formation of the pitted scars of reflux nephropathy.

do not have effective valves to protect the collecting tubules, urine is forced into the parenchyma. Uninfected urine probably causes little harm, but infected urine sets up acute inflammation which is followed by typical deeply pitted scars of *reflux nephropathy* which become more pronounced as the rest of the kidney continues to grow. Compound papillae are usually found at the upper and lower poles of the kidney so it is here that the scarring of reflux nephropathy is most marked (Fig. 6.7).

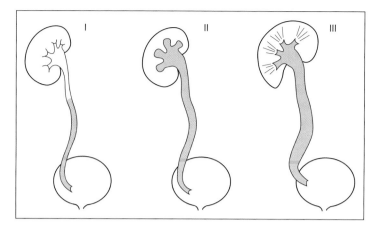

Figure 6.8 Three grades of reflux.

The diagnosis is made by a *micturating cystogram* or ultrasound scan using aerated water in the bladder which shows up on scanning. Three grades of reflux are recognised (Fig. 6.8). In grades I and II, where the reflux is not severe, the urine can usually be kept sterile with a small daily dose of an antimicrobial such as trimethoprim and it is safe to wait for the valve to mature and become competent.

In grade III, where the reflux is gross, it may be impossible to keep the urine sterile, or there is re-peated breakthrough infection, and it may be better to perform an operation to prevent reflux. The most simple of these is to inject a small amount of collagen paste through a cystoscope under the mucosa of the ureteric orifice to change its opening into a crescent (Fig. 6.9). When the ureters are vastly dilated it may be necessary to reimplant the ureter through a long tunnel between the urothelium and muscle of the wall of the bladder (Fig. 6.10).

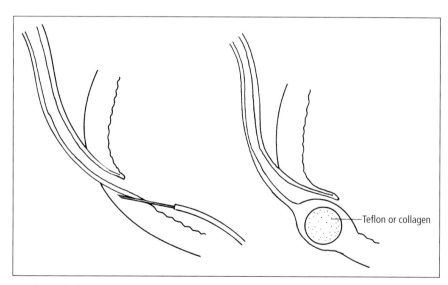

Figure 6.9 A blob of Teflon paste or collagen is injected under the urothelium of the ureteric orifice.

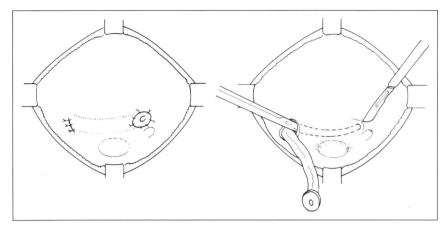

Figure 6.10 Reimplantation of the ureter using Cohen's method.

Complications of urinary tract infection

Acute renal failure

Whether blood- or urine-borne the immediate effect on the parenchyma is like inflammation anywhere else: the kidney becomes hyperaemic, swollen and may lose its function.

Oedema: The patient has pain in the loin and the kidney is tender on palpation. The outline of the kidney and border of the psoas muscle are made fuzzy by oedema, which compresses the necks of the calices (Fig. 6.11).

Loss of function: The intravenous urogram (IVU) may show no excretion of contrast. A dimercapto succinic acid (DMSA) renogram shows no uptake

of isotope in one or more pyramids. There may still be complete recovery (Fig. 6.12).

In acute renal failure, there is an abrupt deterioration in renal function, which is reversible over a period of days or weeks. The aetiologies of acute renal failure are typically classified into pre-renal, post-renal or renal parenchymal causes (discussed in further detail in Chapter 11). Post-renal failure normally results from obstruction of the urinary tract at any point from the renal calyces to the urethra. Some causes of post-renal obstruction include renal/ureteric calculi disease, transitional cell carcinoma causing ureteric obstruction, bladder

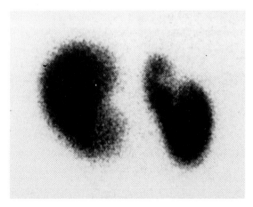

Figure 6.12 DMSA renogram in acute infection showing lack of uptake of the isotope in a pyramid of the left kidney. Courtesy of Dr Neil Garvie.

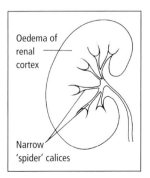

Oedema of renal cortex

Narrow 'spider' calices

Figure 6.11 IVU in acute infection.

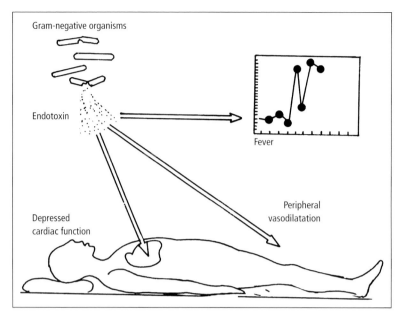

Figure 6.13 Gram-negative septicaemia.

outlet obstruction from an enlarged prostate, urethral strictures and iatrogenic causes such as a blocked urethral catheter.

Obstruction to the urinary tract will predispose to upper urinary tract infections/pyelonephritis. Patients with upper urinary tract infections can develop septicaemia if microorganisms escape from the urinary tract into the bloodstream.

Septicaemia

The most serious of all the complications of acute urinary tract infection is septicaemia. There is only a very thin layer of tissue between the blood vessels of the kidney and the lumen of the urinary tract, and any increase of pressure in the lumen may force microorganisms into the blood stream.

Pathology of gram-negative septicaemia

The organisms most likely to reach the bloodstream are Gram-negative bacilli, which contain *lipid-A endotoxin*. This releases *kinins* which:
• make small blood vessels dilate and become leaky;

• depress the function of the cardiac muscle; and
• stimulate the hypothalamus to cause fever.

Gram-negative septicaemia may occur after any urological operation without warning. There is at first a brief warning stage when the peripheral circulation is dilated, the patient has rigors, fever and a bounding pulse. The face and limbs are flushed and warm. Within half an hour this picture alters dramatically. The blood pressure falls to an unrecordable level. There is vasoconstriction of peripheral vessels and the limbs are cold: the patient looks as though he has suffered a myocardial infarct (Fig. 6.13).

Management
You have no time to lose. Summon help from the team in the Intensive Therapy Unit. Confirm the diagnosis by getting a needle into a vein while you still can find one (which may not be easy). Send blood for culture. Through the same needle inject a massive dose of the most appropriate antibiotic. The choice of antibiotic may be obvious from the preoperative cultures of the urine, but if there is no bacteriological information, ask your colleagues in the hospital microbiology department to advise

you as to the most likely cause of septicaemia and the most appropriate antibiotic.

Set up a saline infusion. Insert a central venous catheter to monitor the pressure in the right heart and then give enough plasma-expander to return the central venous pressure to normal. This may need 5 or 10 L of fluid, and unless the central pressure is carefully monitored you may overload the heart.

Improvement usually takes place within 1 hour, and within 2 hours the peripheral vessels have recovered their tone and the lost fluid begins to return to the circulation. There is now a theoretical risk of overloading the circulation and precipitating heart failure. Usually natural diuresis quickly gets rid of the surplus fluid, but a diuretic is sometimes needed.

When the patient has been resuscitated the *underlying urological problem* can be considered. Any localised pocket of infected urine must be drained, e.g. by percutaneous nephrostomy, emptying the bladder or draining an abscess.

Stone

Stones can form within weeks of an episode of infection. They may form upon a sloughed papilla (see p. 64) or bacterial debris in the urinary tract (Fig. 6.14). Infection with a urea-splitting organism such as *Proteus mirabilis* promotes the formation of a stone.

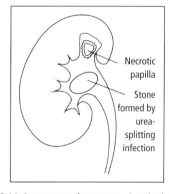

Figure 6.14 Stones may form on a sloughed papilla or bacterial debris.

Suppuration renal carbuncle

Blood-borne infection of the renal parenchyma begins as a collection of little abscesses which coalesce into a collection of pus. In the days before antibiotics staphylococci from a boil in the skin were the usual organisms (Fig. 6.15). Today it is usually *E. coli* from the urinary tract in people who are ill for some other reason, e.g. diabetes mellitus, or immunosuppression. Clinically the patient has a high fever and a swollen, tender kidney. When the infection is confined to the parenchyma there may be no pus cells or organisms in the urine. The X-rays show a soft tissue mass, and in the ultrasound and computed tomography (CT) scans the appearances may be confused with carcinoma. Clinical suspicion will suggest the right diagnosis, and it is confirmed by aspirating pus from the abscess. With effective antibiotic treatment these parenchymal abscesses usually resolve, with a surprising absence of scarring. Diagnosed late, the carbuncle may burst into the perinephric fat forming a perinephric abscess pointing in the loin through the lumbar triangle of Petit, where it is easily drained.

Granulomas

Tuberculosis

At present time, tuberculosis remains a serious problem. The emergence of multi-drug resistant tuberculosis is proving to be a new challenge to physicians worldwide, and for this reason, newer, more effective drugs against *Mycobacterium tuberculosis* will very likely be needed in the future.

The organism is usually transmitted airborne and is initially inhaled into the lungs, where it establishes infection. This is known as primary tuberculosis. Within 1 hour of pulmonary infection, the bacilli are able to infiltrate the pulmonary lymphatics and thus enter the bloodstream. Although the initial numbers of these bacilli are not high, there is now a small risk of the patient developing extra-pulmonary TB by the process of seeding.

In the urinary tract, one of two things may happen: disseminated bacilli that become lodged in

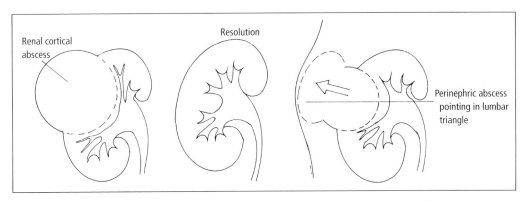

Figure 6.15 Blood-borne infection may give rise to cortical infection which may resolve or proceed to an abscess.

the renal cortex from the bloodstream may be destroyed by normal host tissue resistance and no infection is established. However, if the bacilli are of sufficient numbers and virulence, an infective focus may be established (Fig. 6.16). At this stage patients may notice frequency of micturition and haematuria. The IVU may show an irregularity in a renal papilla which can be easy to overlook.

Later the abscess in the papilla enlarges, grows out to involve the rest of the pyramid, and may calcify (Fig. 6.17). The inflammation may narrow the neck of one or more calices which then fill with calcified debris (Fig. 6.18) and eventually the entire kidney can be converted into a bag of calcified caseation tissue which has a striking appearance in the plain X-ray — *cement kidney* (Fig. 6.19).

From the kidney the infection spreads down the ureter to the bladder. The ureter becomes stiff,

oedematous and shortened so that the ureteric orifice is pulled up to give the appearance of a golf-hole (Fig. 6.20). Later on, as antituberculous chemotherapy begins to work and the unsuspected granulomas in the wall of the ureter heal up, the ureter may become narrowed by scarring to cause hydronephrosis (Fig. 6.21).

In the bladder the early phase of tuberculosis may cause oedema, ulceration or inflammatory polypi resembling a tumour on cystoscopy. Biopsy shows the characteristic tubercles, giant cells and acid-fast bacilli. The lesions in the bladder rapidly heal with treatment, but as with the ureter, scarring may cause the bladder to shrink with the result that the patient may have severe frequency of micturition.

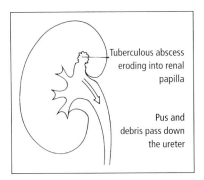

Figure 6.16 Tuberculous abscess in a renal papilla.

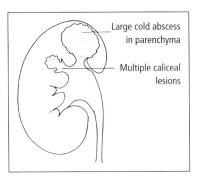

Figure 6.17 Extension of the tuberculous abscess to the calix.

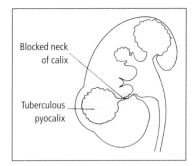

Figure 6.18 Multiple tuberculous pyocalices.

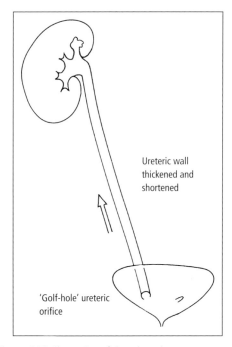

Figure 6.20 Shortening of the tuberculous ureter.

Diagnosis

It needs suspicion to diagnose genitourinary tuberculosis. One good rule is to insist that every patient with pus in the urine, not explained by bacterial infection, must have tuberculosis excluded. The diagnosis of tuberculosis is not easy to make because *Mycobacterium* are notoriously slow growing and cultures of this bacteria take up to six weeks to be ready. Diagnosis may be made on the basis of the following investigations:

Early morning urine specimens (three in total) are stained for acid and alcohol-fast bacilli (AAFB) using the Ziehl-Nielsen (ZN) stain or auramine and UV light. Urine is then tested for tuberculosis by incubating on Lowenstein-Jensen (solid) or Bectan-Dickinson (liquid) cultures. Any positive growths will require a further month before antibiotic sensitivities can be determined.

Fresh tissue biopsies from the affected area of the urinary tract can be used for cultures if the above tests do not yield any results.

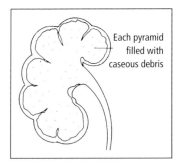

Figure 6.19 The cement kidney.

Treatment

Tuberculosis is a systemic disease. The patient often has active disease in the chest. The disease must be notified so that contacts can be traced. In practice this means you should summon the help of a colleague, usually a chest physician, who can treat the whole patient and will be expert in the dosage and details of combination chemotherapy. Anti-tuberculous treatment typically consists of once daily rifampicin 600 mg (reduced to 450 mg if body weight is less than 55 kg) and isoniazid 300 mg for a total of 6 months. In combination to the above, pyrazinamide 2 g daily is administered for the first 2 months of treatment. Pyridoxine 10 mg is given daily to reduce the risk of isoniazid-induced poly-neuropathy. Second-line treatments can include ethambutol and streptomycin. Today more cases are being found where the mycobacteria are resistant to these first-line antibiotics: another reason for getting expert help.

This does not mean that the urologist has handed over his or her responsibilities: each case

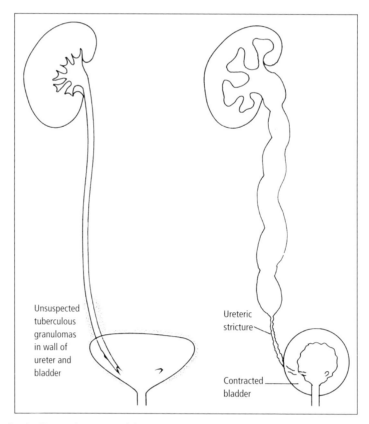

Figure 6.21 Healing leading to obstruction of the ureter.

must be carefully followed up. With small lesions in one or two renal papillae one expects a complete resolution with, at worst, a fleck of calcification to mark the site of the tuberculous granuloma. Healing may lead to stenosis of the ureter and to detect this the intravenous urogram (IVU) or ultrasound must be repeated within 2 weeks of starting treatment. Early stenosis of the ureter may be prevented by means of a double-J splint for a few weeks, and so long as the sensitivity of the mycobacteria is certain and antibiotics are being given, steroids may assist in the prevention of scarring.

If a stricture does form up near the renal pelvis a pyeloplasty may be performed. When the narrowing is near the bladder the ureter may need to be reimplanted. If the entire length of the ureter is stenosed, it can be replaced with ileum. A contracted bladder can be enlarged by one or other types of cystoplasty.

Unfortunately patients often come up at a stage when the kidney is too badly affected to recover useful function: in these cases, after preliminary treatment with antibiotics nephrectomy should be performed. Thanks to the efficacy of modern chemotherapy there is no longer any need to remove the ureter as well.

In males urinary tuberculosis may be accompanied by tuberculosis of the prostate, seminal vesicles, epididymes and vasa deferentia. In women there may be involvement of the fallopian tubes and uterus.

Xanthogranuloma

This is a rare disorder that can give rise to granulomas and renal masses in children. The patient usually has pyrexia, loin pain, urinary tract infection and weight loss. This can occur around a renal calculus usually in association with *Proteus mirabilis*

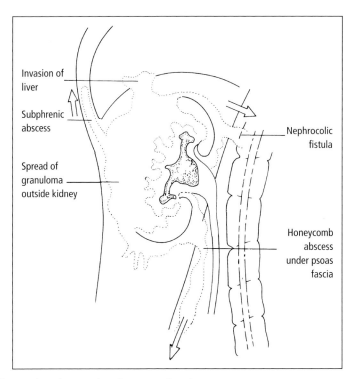

Figure 6.22 Xanthogranuloma burrows into the surrounding tissues.

infection. Macroscopically, the renal mass consists of a firm, yellow and lobulated tissue, which resembles renal cell carcinoma. However, microscopically, histiocyte cells are stuffed with lipid. The inflammation burrows into the tissues around the kidney (Fig. 6.22) as well as adjacent viscera, e.g. liver, colon and duodenum. Antibiotics alone are insufficient for treatment. Xanthogranulomas are traditionally managed with surgical excision.

Malacoplakia

Another curious granuloma of the urinary tract gives rise to multiple abscesses and dense fibrosis. In the bladder and ureter it produces soft brown plaques which bleed easily, and may cause obstruction. It may respond to a prolonged course of trimethoprim.

Brucellosis

Brucellosis is a zoonotic disease that may cause granulomatosis in the human kidney. The *Brucella* family is quite varied and there are subspecies that can be found in farm and household domesticated animals (cattle – *Brucella abortus*; sheep – *B. ovis*; dogs – *B. canis*). They are small gram-negative coccobacilli that are non-motile.

The routes of transmission include direct contact with infected animals or their secretions through cuts and abrasions on the skin, ingestion of unpasteurised dairy products or inhalation of infectious aerosols. Renal complications are rare, however, interstitial nephritis, glomerulonephritis and IgA nephropathy have been previously reported. Chronic renal abscess formation may indeed mimic tuberculotic granulomas. Epididymo-orchitis occurs in up to 20% of men with brucellosis.

Interstitial nephritis, pyelonephritis, papillary necrosis

A wide variety of causes lead to a spectrum of changes in the kidney which vary from diffuse

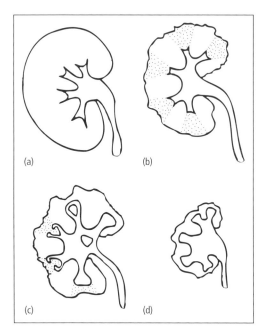

Figure 6.23 Spectrum of changes in pyelonephritis.

scarring throughout the renal parenchyma – *interstitial nephritis* to – at the other end, necrosis of entire renal papillae, which may become completely detached – *papillary necrosis* (Fig. 6.23). Among these causes are:

1 *Infection:* Severe infection, particularly when combined with obstruction, can lead to interstitial nephritis, and in severe cases, to necrosis of the papilla especially when there is obstruction or some other underlying disorder such as diabetes mellitus.

2 *Analgesic abuse:* There have been epidemics in which whole populations have taken to consuming large amounts of aspirin, phenacitin and similar analgesic medications: examples include the housewives of Newcastle (Australia), the watchmakers of Switzerland, and the motorcycle workers of Husqvarna in Sweden. They show every combination of interstitial nephritis and papillary necrosis.

3 *Balkan nephropathy:* In isolated villages in the Balkans epidemics occur in which large numbers of people develop interstitial nephritis and papillary necrosis, probably caused by a herb, see below.

4 *Chinese herbal sliming medicines:* Belgian ladies attending a fashionable slimming clinic were given an extract of *Aristolochia fang-ji* by mistake. Many developed renal failure, and a few survivors went on to develop multifocal cancer. It has been suggested that perhaps a similar herb, *Aristolochia clematis*, may be responsible for Balkan nephropathy (see above).

5 *Gout and nephrocalcinosis:* The sharp needles of uric acid found in *gout*, and crystals of calcium salts found in *nephrocalcinosis* are deposited in and around the renal tubules and may provoke scarring similar to interstitial nephritis.

Clinical features

Whatever the cause, the clinical features of interstitial nephritis are similar. There is loss of protein and progressive failure of the function, at first of the renal tubules, and later of the glomeruli. In severe cases the sloughed renal papillae may become detached and pass down the ureter (causing obstruction) or remain and calcify in the kidney, to form a stone with a typically radiolucent centre (Fig. 6.24). Many of these patients come to dialysis, and years later, the survivors are prone to develop multifocal transitional cell cancer involving the renal pelvis and calices.

Hydatid disease

The tapeworm *Echinococcus granulosus* normally lives in sheep. Dogs may eat uncooked sheep offal containing the worms, which thrive inside the dog, and shed eggs which collect on the dog's fur. Children fondle the dogs, forget to wash their hands, and swallow the ova. The eggs hatch out, and the worms burrow through the wall of the child's gut to reach the liver and kidney where they grow, multiply and form collections of cysts. The cysts are multilocular. Their walls are more or less calcified, and the appearances are easily mistaken for cancer on ultrasound or CT scanning (Fig. 6.25). An immunoassay for a specific circulating antigen confirms the diagnosis. If, by mistake,

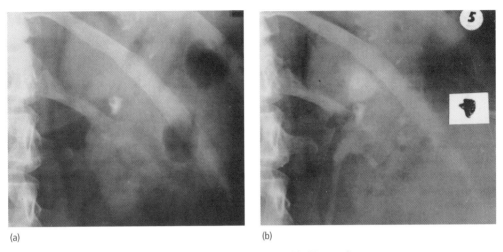

(a)   (b)

Figure 6.24 Calcification on a dead papilla forming a stone which is blocking a calix.

the fluid inside the hydatid cyst is aspirated it will be found to be full of little hooklets (Fig. 6.26) but aspiration is avoided because it may spread the disease as well as precipitate an acute allergic attack.

After a course of *albendazole* the affected kidney should be removed, taking great care not to spill the cysts. The kidney is approached through the loin and the wound protected with packs soaked in 1% formalin or hypertonic saline. The biggest cysts are then aspirated, and the fluid replaced with 1% formalin or hypertonic saline, reaspirated, and only when there is no risk of the kidney bursting, is it removed *en bloc*. If the tiny tapeworms inside the cysts are spilt they give rise to local recurrence which may be inoperable.

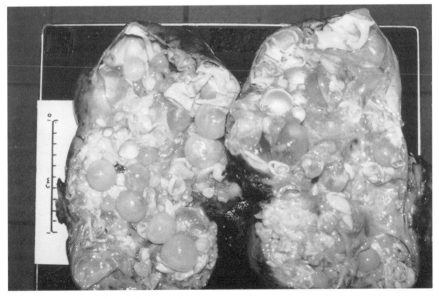

Figure 6.25 Multiple hydatid cysts in a human kidney.

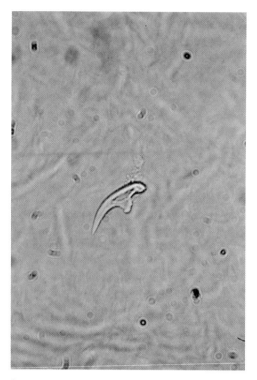

Figure 6.26 Hooklet in fluid aspirated from a hydatid cyst.

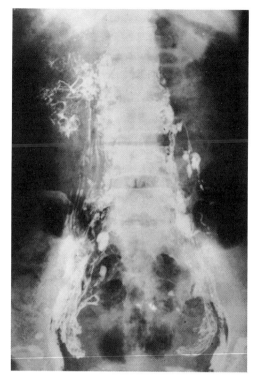

Figure 6.27 Lymphangiogram and retrograde urogram showing connection with lymphatics of the kidney, in a case of chyluria.

Chyluria

The passage of protein-rich fluid with chyle or lymphatic fluid is known as chyluria. This is frequently noted by the patient by the presence of milky white urine. This condition is usually attributed to a lymphatic urinary fistula caused by obstruction of the renal lymphatics, resulting in forniceal rupture and leakage. Occasionally, chyluria may be caused by filariasis infestation, trauma, tuberculosis or retroperitoneal tumours. In the Far East, fistula formation between the perirenal lymphatics and the renal pelvis may be caused by infestation with the roundworm *Wuchereria bancroftii*, which is transmitted by mosquitoes (Fig. 6.27).

The management of chyluria is usually conservative as it tends to resolve spontaneously. However, in persistent and severe proteinuria, silver nitrate or hypertonic saline can be injected through a ureteric catheter to seal off the communications. If this fails, the kidney may be dissected from the lymphatics, which must all be carefully ligated.

Chapter 7

Urinary calculi

Operations for the stone were well known in the time of Hippocrates, whose Oath enjoined young doctors to leave 'cutting for the stone' to those who were properly trained to do it. The incidence of stone varies in different populations. In the West there has been a steady rise in the incidence of calculi in the kidney and ureter, interrupted only by two World Wars, from which it is argued that stones reflect affluence and overfeeding with re-fined sugar and protein. Stones are more common in those whose work causes them to become de-hydrated and form more concentrated urine. It is probable that the incidence of bladder stones in children in underdeveloped countries is a mani-festation of infantile diarrhoea diseases and dehy-dration.

A stone consists of crystalline material arranged in layers on an organic scaffold like ferroconcrete or fibreglass (Fig. 7.1). We know little about the organic scaffold, but a lot about the formation of the crystals.

Salt added to water continues to dissolve until no more will do so: this is the saturation concen-tration, which is measured by the solubility prod-uct of the concentration of ions making up the salt (Fig. 7.2). In urine a metastable solution forms

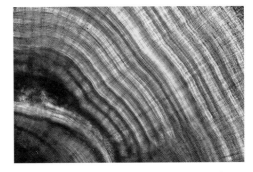

Figure 7.1 Cross section of a stone showing its lamina-tions.

which does not precipitate crystals, even though the saturation concentration has been exceeded, unless the solution is left undisturbed for a long time, or is seeded with a nucleus on which stones

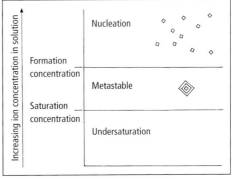

Figure 7.2 Increasing ion concentration in a fluid such as urine.

Lecture Notes: Urology, 6th edition. By John Blandy and Amir Kaisary. Published 2009 by Blackwell Publishing. ISBN: 978-1-4051-2270-2.

can precipitate. If the concentration exceeds that of the metastable region, crystals precipitate to make their own nuclei – nucleation. Human urine is always metastable with respect to the main crystalline components of stones, calcium and oxalate.

The metastable state is influenced by temperature, the presence of colloids, the rate of flow of the urine, the concentration of the solutes and the presence of anything which can act as a nucleus, e.g. dead papillae, necrotic carcinoma, a non-absorbable suture, a fragment of catheter, or a previously existing fragment of stone (Fig. 7.3).

The pH of the urine may be important in the formation of calculi: magnesium ammonium phosphate is insoluble in alkaline urine, and is precipitated by infection with *Proteus mirabilis* and other urea-splitting organisms. Uric acid is insoluble in acid urine, but may dissolve if the urine is made alkaline.

All crystals prefer to be undisturbed if they are to grow, so calculi tend to form wherever there is stagnant urine, as in a ureterocele, a diverticulum, a hydronephrosis or a chronically obstructed bladder.

Supersaturation stones

The best examples of supersaturation stones are cystine and uric acid.

Cystine

In cystinuria there is a congenital (Mendelian recessive) defect in the enzymes necessary for the transport of cystine, ornithine, arginine and lysine in the proximal tubule (see p. 45). Homozygotes pass about 1 g/24 h, heterozygotes about 0.5 g. Cystine is more soluble in alkaline urine: penicillamine produces a soluble penicillamine–cysteine molecule.

Uric acid

Uric acid is a weak acid and is only half-ionised in urine of pH 5.75. A much greater proportion

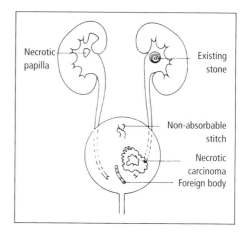

Figure 7.3 Many things can act as a nucleus for stone formation.

is found in a soluble ionised form in the alkaline urine. If the urine is allowed to become acid, most of it will be precipitated. An excess of uric acid occurs when there is a primary defect of metabolism of uric acid (as in gout) or rapid catabolism of protein, e.g. after cancer chemotherapy. Uric acid stones occur whenever the urine is very concentrated and very acid, as is seen in dehydration and in patients with ulcerative colitis and ileostomies. In addition, the distal tubules in some patients are not able to form alkaline urine, and thus they tend to have uric acid stones.

Treatment consists of encouraging a large water intake, together with bicarbonate to keep the urine alkaline, and perhaps allopurinol to inhibit xanthine oxidase and prevent the formation of uric acid.

Calcium stones

Most non-infective stones are made of calcium oxalate and/or calcium phosphate.

Oxalate

Primary (hepatic) oxaluria

An excess of oxalate is formed in primary hyperoxaluria, because of an inherited liver enzyme

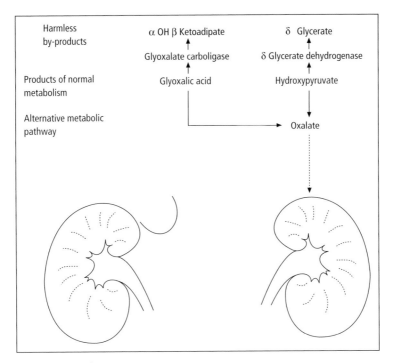

Figure 7.4 Primary or hepatic oxaluria.

deficiency (either of glyoxalate carboligase, or gamma-glycerate dehydrogenase) leading to an excess of oxalate in the urine which precipitates in the collecting tubules and eventually leads to renal failure (Fig. 7.4). Unfortunately, a transplanted kidney suffers the same fate, but a combined liver and kidney transplant can be successful.

Secondary (ileal) oxaluria

Hyperoxaluria also occurs in diseases of the terminal ileum where bile acids are normally absorbed. If bile acids are not reabsorbed and recycled in the liver to be added to bile, then dietary fat cannot be emulsified, and remains in the bowel where it forms an insoluble soap with dietary calcium (Fig. 7.5). This in turn leaves an excess of dietary oxalate which is absorbed, excreted in the urine, and forms a stone. This type of hyperoxaluria may be prevented by giving cholestyramine (which binds the oxalate in the gut) and by avoid-

ing food rich in oxalate such as tea, chocolate, coffee, spinach and rhubarb.

Hypercalciuria

An excess of calcium in the urine (i.e. >350 mg/24 h in males, >300 mg/24 h in females) may be a cause of stones in some males. These are of three types:

1 Renal, where there is decreased renal tubular reabsorption of calcium. Little can be done about this.

2 Absorptive, where too much calcium is absorbed from the bowel. Many types of treatment were formerly given to diminish this, e.g. cellulose phosphate was given to precipitate calcium salts in the bowel: patients were advised to give up milk products as well as all those rich in oxalate. In addition, magnesium salts were given to try to keep calcium particles in suspension in the urine. In fact, all these treatments were ineffective and

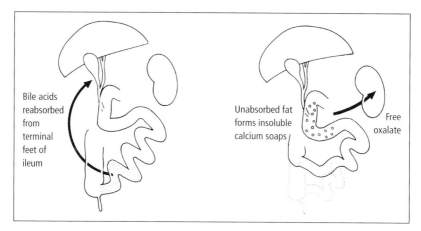

Figure 7.5 Ileal oxaluria.

it is far more important to keep the urine dilute by drinking plenty of water, and perhaps encourage this with a small dose of a diuretic such as frusemide.

3 Resorptive hypercalciuria, where an excess of calcium is absorbed from the bones, depends on the function of the parathyroid glands.

Most of the calcium in the blood is bound to protein; only a small fraction is in solution, and of this an even smaller part is ionised. The product of the ions $[Ca \times PO_4]$ is kept constant. If $[Ca]$ is increased, then $[PO_4]$ must fall, and vice versa. Parathyroid hormone encourages osteoclasts to dissolve bone and release calcium into the blood: the output of the hormone is regulated by the concentration of ionised $[Ca]$. There are three types of hyperparathyroidism as follows.

Primary hyperparathyroidism

For no known reason, the parathyroid glands start to secrete more parathyroid hormone than is needed with the result that calcium is reabsorbed from the skeleton and added to the blood. The plasma $[Ca]$ rises and the plasma $[PO_4]$ has to fall. The excess calcium enters the urine where it precipitates in the renal tubules as one form of

nephrocalcinosis, or forms a stone in the renal tract (Fig. 7.6).

The diagnosis of primary hyperparathyroidism is usually made by the chance finding of an elevated $[Ca]$ in the course of a routine blood test or in the investigation of a patient with a stone. It is very rare to find the classical changes of osteitis fibrosa cystica where massive collections of osteoclasts cause cystic cavities in bones and sometimes a pathological fracture. The finding of elevated plasma $[Ca]$ must always be double checked, and if confirmed, then the plasma parathyroid hormone is measured by radioimmunoassay.

Secondary hyperparathyroidism

In chronic renal failure, phosphate is one of the metabolic products that is not adequately excreted; so, the plasma $[PO_4]$ rises, and the $[Ca]$ has to fall. The $[Ca]$ is precipitated in soft tissues as heterotopic calcification where it may cause joint stiffness and deafness. The parathyroids respond to the lowered $[Ca]$ by secreting more parathyroid hormone, and all four glands become hyperplastic. Secondary hyperparathyroidism is still seen in patients undergoing dialysis for renal failure, but can largely be prevented by large doses of vitamin

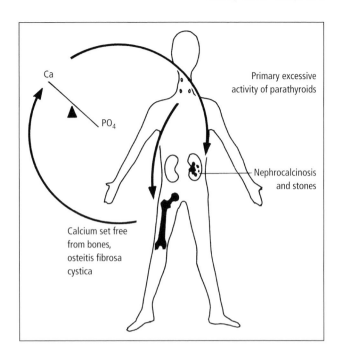

Figure 7.6 Primary hyperparathyroidism.

D which encourage the absorption of calcium from the bowel (Fig. 7.7).

Tertiary hyperparathyroidism

Here the overactive parathyroid glands seem not to know when to stop and in spite of extra vitamin D, keep on putting out far more parathyroid hormone than is needed to maintain a constant [Ca]. When this occurs, they must be removed.

Parathyroidectomy

The four parathyroid glands are each about the size of a pea and lie behind and buried in the lateral lobes of the thyroid gland near the superior and inferior thyroid arteries (Fig. 7.8). Primary hyperparathyroidism may be caused by an adenoma in one gland or hyperplasia of all four. The glands are localised by subtraction of radioisotope scans, and at operation all four glands are confirmed by biopsy and frozen section. Occasionally, a 'missing' parathyroid gland is found in the mediastinum.

Formation of renal calculi

Tiny spheres of calcium phosphate are often found in normal collecting ducts – Carr's concretions. Collections of these concretions gather near the tip of a papilla to form shining plaques easily seen with a nephroscope – Randall's plaques. When these become detached, they may act as a nucleus for further stone formation (Fig. 7.9). A similar nucleus is formed by a necrotic renal papilla. From then on, the stone continues to grow as layer after layer of calcium salts, together with a protein matrix, is laid down.

Investigation of a calculus

Where is the stone, and is it likely to do any harm?

An intravenous urogram (IVU) or a computed tomography (CT) IVU will usually show where the stone is situated, and whether it is likely to get stuck and cause obstruction. The exceptions are those made of uric acid and cystine. Stones made of uric acid are completely radiolucent, and do not

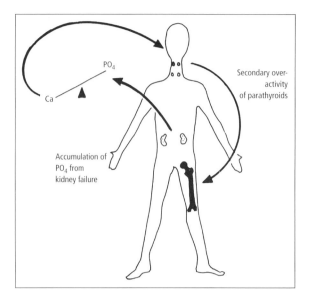

Figure 7.7 Secondary hyperparathyroidism.

show in a plain radiograph, but they do cast an acoustic shadow on ultrasound scan and show up in a CT scan. Stones made of cystine are faintly radio-opaque because of their sulphur content, and are always easily located with ultrasound or CT scan. A combination of CT IVU is the best investigation when a stone is suspected.

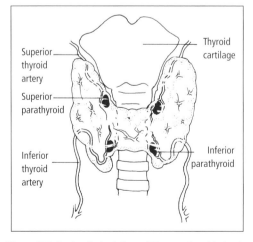

Figure 7.8 Anatomical relations of the parathyroid glands.

What is the cause of the stone, and can it be prevented?

Hyperparathyroidism must be ruled out by measuring the plasma [Ca]. The urine should be checked for infection especially with urea-splitting organisms. The whole state of the urinary tract needs to be examined for possible collections of stagnant urine, and one must always consider the possibility that the stone may have formed on a non-absorbable suture or other foreign body.

Management of a renal stone

As a general rule the normal ureter will allow a stone to pass if it is less than 5 mm in diameter. Stones larger than this are likely to get stuck and should usually be removed.

When a stone is stuck it causes obstruction, but this rarely remains complete for very long, and the urine soon finds its way past the stone. If the urine also happens to be infected there is a risk that back-pressure will cause septicaemia and/or obstructive nephropathy so then it is urgently necessary to overcome the obstruction either by an emergency percutaneous nephrostomy or by passing a double-J splint from below. The infection cannot usually be eradicated if a stone

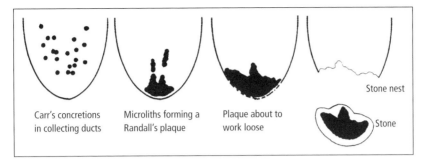

Figure 7.9 Formation of calculus in a renal papilla.

is present because it shields microorganisms from antibiotics. Urea-splitting organisms will precipitate layers of magnesium ammonium phosphate (apatite) on any existing stone.

Methods for removing stones

Extracorporeal shock wave lithotripsy

Shock waves travel through water. Different types of lithotriptors generate shock waves, and focus them on the stone by means of X-rays or ultrasonic scanners. The shock waves break the stone up into fragments small enough to pass down the ureter.

Many different types of lithotriptors are available, differing in the method by which the shock wave is generated and the stone is localised. To generate the shock wave some use a spark plug, others an array of piezoceramic shock emitters (Fig. 7.10). Some localise the stone with ultrasound, others use X-rays.

However, the stone is broken up, the little fragments have to go down the ureter. There, they may

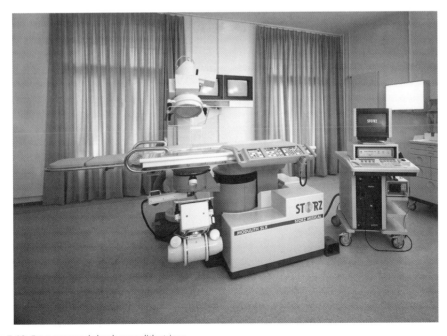

Figure 7.10 Extracorporeal shock wave lithotripsy.

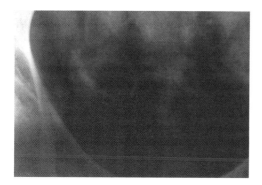

Figure 7.11 Steinstrasse – collection of fragments held up in the lower ureter after ESWL.

cause temporary obstruction – the *steinstrasse* – and diclofenac may be needed for ureteric colic (Fig. 7.11) but with a large fluid throughput the steinstrasse usually clears within a few days. Alpha-blockers help these little particles of stone to pass spontaneously.

It may be necessary to repeat the lithotripsy several times, according to the density of the stones. For larger stones extracorporeal shock wave lithotripsy (ESWL) is often combined with percutaneous nephrolithotomy (PCNL).

Percutaneous nephrolithotomy

After placing a needle under X-ray or ultrasound control into the renal pelvis, a guidewire is passed, and the needle withdrawn. A series of dilators of increasing size are then passed over the guidewire

until a track has been made into the kidney big enough to admit a working sheath, through which instruments can be passed (Fig. 7.12). The stone is now examined with a nephroscope, and broken up with one of several ingenious gadgets: one emits a stream of sparks which cracks the stone; another does the same thing with a Q-switched laser; a third grinds the stone to powder with a toothed cylinder oscillated at ultrasonic frequency; and a fourth uses a miniature jackhammer to break up the stone. Some probes are hollowed so that the fragments can be sucked out while the stone is being broken up. A variety of forceps are available to pick out the bits (Fig. 7.13).

Double-J ureteric stent

To help the ureter to dilate, and encourage the passage of the fragments of stone after ESWL, a double-J stent is often passed up the ureter over a guidewire introduced through a flexible or rigid cystoscope (Fig. 7.14). The double-J splint can be left in for several weeks, but there is a risk that the double-J splint may itself act as a nucleus for stone formation, and strict precautions have to be taken to follow the patient up and make sure the stent is retrieved within a reasonable time.

Ureteroscopy

A ureteroscope, rigid or flexible, may be passed up the ureter to break up and remove small stones

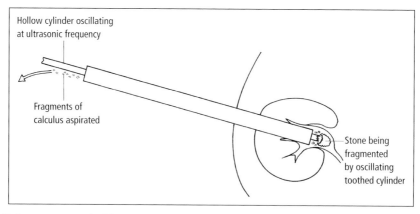

Figure 7.12 Percutaneous nephrolithotomy.

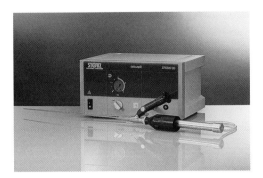

Figure 7.13 Storz ultrasonic lithotriptor.

that are stuck in the ureter: miniature versions of the Q-switched laser and jackhammer are available for this procedure (Fig. 7.15).

Stones in common sites

Stone in a calix

Caliceal stones seldom cause any trouble and can as a rule be safely kept under observation. Very

occasionally, they seem to cause pain and may be fragmented by ESWL.

Stone in the renal pelvis

A stone in the renal pelvis which is more than 5 mm in diameter will probably get stuck when it tries to go down the ureter. Some urologists advocate utilising ESWL or PCNL to get rid of the stone before the patient has any symptoms. These renal pelvic stones can cause repeated attacks of renal pain or ureteric colic and haematuria, and may be associated with infection.

Stones in the pelvis used to be removed by open pyelolithotomy. The kidney was approached through the 12th rib tip incision, and mobilised to give access to the renal pelvis, which was opened between stay stitches: the stone was removed, the pelvis closed and the wound closed with a drain (Fig. 7.16). The same procedure can be done laparoscopically.

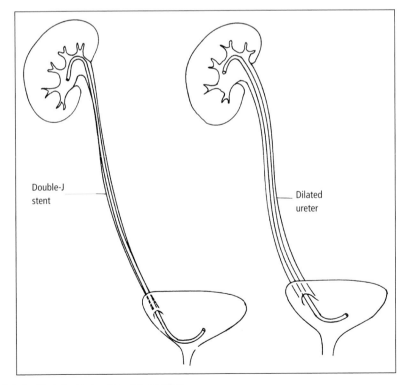

Double-J stent

Dilated ureter

Figure 7.14 A double-J stent helps the ureter to dilate.

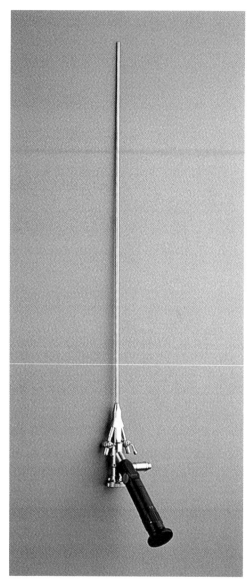

Figure 7.15 Storz ureteroscope.

Staghorn stones

Stones sometimes fill the entire pelvis and nearly all the calices (Fig. 7.17), usually in the presence of *Proteus mirabilis* infection. The body of the stone is usually removed by PCNL while the outlying bits in the calices are broken up with extracorporeal lithotripsy in a series of sessions. This can require

the patient to undergo a long series of operations, even though none of them are very major, and at the end of the day small bits of stone are often left behind. From time to time it is still necessary to perform an open extended pyelolithotomy (Fig. 7.18).

Here the kidney is approached through the loin, fully mobilised, its renal artery taped (for safety) and the bloodless plane between the renal pelvis and parenchyma opened up to allow the parenchyma to be lifted up, after which the pelvis is laid open up from the upper to the lower calix. The stone is then extracted completely, and the kidney confirmed to be clear with an X-ray in situ. The renal pelvis is sewn up and the wound closed with drainage. Again the same operation can be done laparoscopically.

Stones in the ureter

'Little dogs make the most noise'. The pain of a stone in the ureter is excruciating. It comes on suddenly, in waves that make the patient roll and twist to get relief. Extravasation of urine into the retroperitoneal tissues may cause vomiting, and distension of the bowel mimics intestinal obstruction. There may be tenderness over the loin and iliac fossa (Fig. 7.19). A trace of blood is often present in the urine.

Stones less than 5 mm in diameter will usually pass down the ureter on their own, at the expense of several bouts of pain that are usually relieved by diclofenac. Alpha-blockers may help the stone progress steadily. If there is no infection, no operation is indicated but infection calls for an immediate percutaneous nephrostomy.

When the stone is not making progress, is obviously too big, or remains stuck for several weeks, it is removed by ESWL. It can be broken up with an instrument introduced via the ureteroscope, but this carries a risk of injury to the ureter and is used with the utmost caution. Successful retrieval of a stone is more likely in the lower third of the ureter than the upper third.

The classical operation was open ureterolithotomy. Under general anaesthetic a short incision was made over the appropriate part of the ureter,

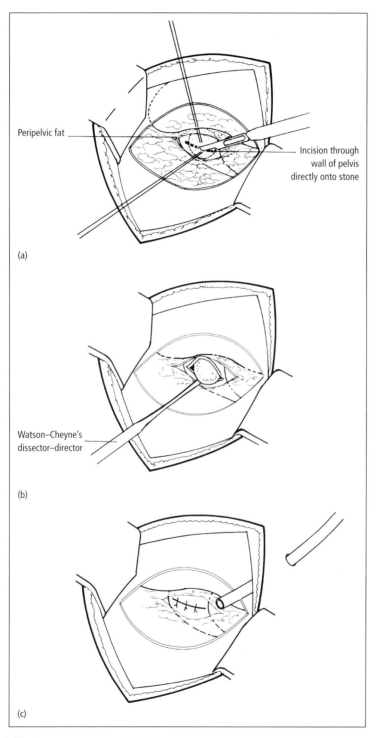

Peripelvic fat

Incision through
wall of pelvis
directly onto stone

(a)

Watson–Cheyne's
dissector–director

(b)

(c)

Figure 7.16 Pyelolithotomy.

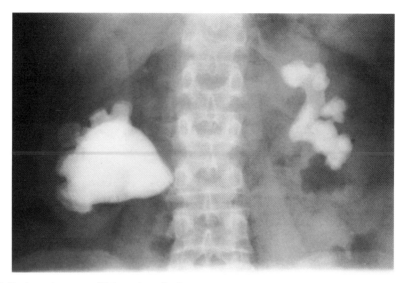

Figure 7.17 Staghorn stones may fill the entire collecting system.

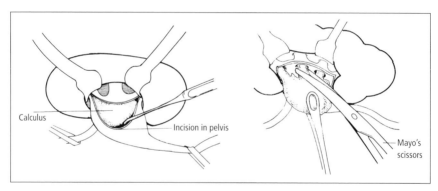

Figure 7.18 Extended pyelolithotomy.

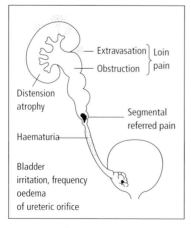

Figure 7.19 Clinical features of a stone in the ureter.

the peritoneum was reflected medially and the stone located with a finger. A short incision in the ureter allowed the stone to be prised out, and the wound was then closed with drainage. Unlike ureteroscopic operations, the incision in the ureter always healed spontaneously, did not need to be sutured and was never followed by a stricture (Fig. 7.20). This procedure may also be done laparoscopically.

Stones in the bladder

A stone that is small enough to pass down the ureter can usually get out of the bladder, and most ureteric stones pass without being noticed.

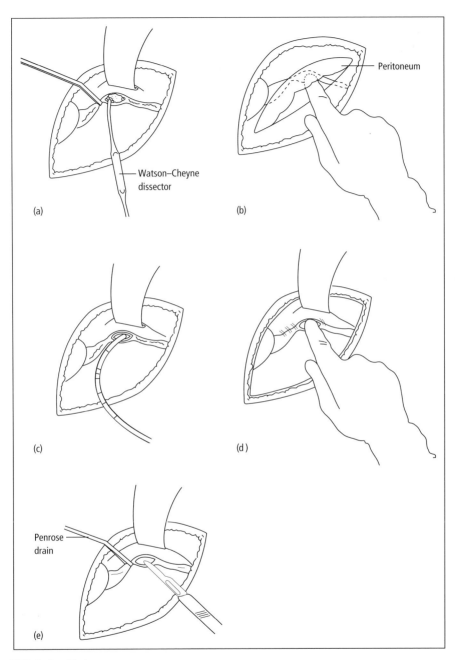

Figure 7.20 Ureterolithotomy.

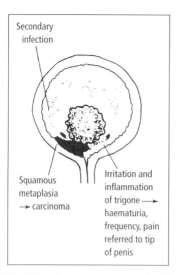

Figure 7.21 Clinical features of a stone in the bladder.

Obstruction to the outflow of the bladder may trap the stones and today, in the West, bladder stones are seen only in elderly men with prostatic obstruction. In women, bladder stones are even more rare and usually formed on a non-absorbable stitch.

The symptoms are those of outflow obstruction without pain or haematuria (Fig. 7.21), but sometimes pain is referred to the tip of the penis, and is made worse by exercise and is relieved by lying down.

Small bladder stones are seen through a resectoscope sheath, broken up with forceps and washed

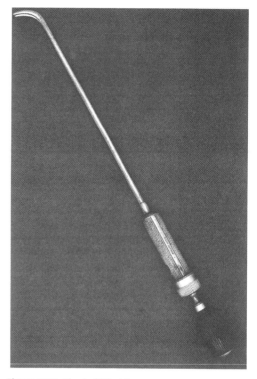

Figure 7.22 Classical lithotrite.

out. Larger ones are crushed with the classical lithotrite (Fig. 7.22), its modern visual counterpart (Fig. 7.23), the Swiss jackhammer or the Q-switched laser.

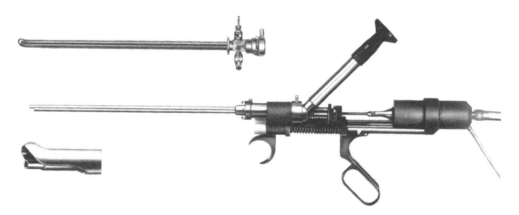

Figure 7.23 Storz ultrasonic lithotriptor. (Courtesy Rimmer Bros, UK Agents for Karl Storz.)

In little boys, and in adults with very large stones that fill the bladder, a suprapubic lithotomy is safer. A short incision is made over the full bladder which is opened between stay sutures and the stone lifted out. The bladder is closed with an indwelling catheter that remains in place for 5–6 days.

Key messages

1 Single stone formers might not require extensive metabolic evaluation but the patient's dietary habits, oral fluid intake and excessive intake of certain foods and medications ought to be recorded.

2 Stone analysis can direct metabolic investigations and save the need for a complete metabolic evaluation.

3 Recurrent stone formers are recommended to undergo a complete metabolic evaluation.

4 Patients should be strongly encouraged to consume fluid enough to produce an average of 1.5–2 L of urine daily.

5 Dietary intake which increases the risk of stone formation includes high protein and low-carbohydrate diet and large doses of vitamin C (>2 g/day).

6 Calcium supplements are safest if taken with diet.

7 Obesity is an independent risk factor for urinary stone formation, particularly in females.

Chapter 8

Neoplasms of the kidney

Embryoma (Wilms' tumour)

Embryoma accounts for 10% of all childhood cancers and is seen in 1:13,000 children. There are two types of which one is inherited: this group is caused by an autosomal dominant with loss of genetic material on chromosome 11. It is associated with aniridia, hemihypertrophy, macroglossia, multicystic disease, neurofibromatosis and adult renal cell cancer.

In the first few months, one particular subgroup has to be distinguished because it behaves almost as though it were benign – *mesoblastic nephroma*. It must be completely excised. One in 10 Wilms' tumours is bilateral. There are two distinct pathological entities – *favourable* and *unfavourable*, according to the amount of undifferentiated tissue that is present. The worst of this is usually *rhabdomyosarcoma*. Embryomas spread both by direct invasion into the adjacent muscle and bowel as well as by the bloodstream to the lungs. Erosion of the renal pelvis occurs relatively late, so that when *haematuria* occurs the prognosis is bad. The International Union Against Cancer (UICC) system of staging is represented in Fig. 8.1.

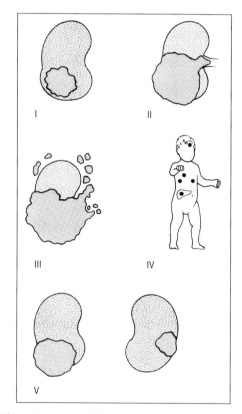

Figure 8.1 Stages of Wilms' tumour.

Lecture Notes: Urology, 6th edition. By John Blandy and Amir Kaisary. Published 2009 by Blackwell Publishing. ISBN: 978-1-4051-2270-2.

Clinical features

'A big lump in a wasted baby'

A mother bathing her baby notices a lump: this is the classical presentation (Fig. 8.2), but these tumours may present with pain and haematuria, as well as hypertension, fever and a raised red or white cell count. Ultrasound is the first investigation, followed by computed tomography (CT) scanning, even if this may require a general anaesthetic. In practice, the differential diagnosis is from *neuroblastoma*, which usually has speckled calcification, and displaces the kidney downwards.

Management

Today, thanks to a combination of radical surgery and chemotherapy one can expect 96% 4-year survival in stage I disease, and even in stage III disease, so long as the histology is 'favourable' the survival is >87%. But to achieve these results requires expert management by a dedicated team. Every child with a Wilms' tumour deserves to be referred to a specialised centre regularly auditing its results in trials of the latest protocols. It is not for the occasional surgeon in a small hospital. One such protocol calls for a 5-day course of actinomycin D followed by laparotomy at which the renal vessels are tied before the tumour is handled, and the op-

posite kidney is carefully examined. The kidney is then removed radically, with a wide margin. Postoperatively vincristine is given. Radiotherapy is *not* necessary in stage I tumours. It is always given in stage III. Its role in stage II is still under review.

Renal cell cancer – Grawitz tumour (hypernephroma)

Grawitz tumour is a tumour of grandfathers (Fig. 8.3). It is rare before puberty, and less common in females. It may be associated with cadmium pollution. More and more new tumours are now being found by ultrasound scanning of patients who have been on long-term renal dialysis. It is associated with the *von Hippel–Lindau syndrome*, i.e. angiomas in the cerebellum and retina and cysts in the liver and pancreas.

Pathology

Many healthy adults have small 'adenomas' in their kidneys, which arise from the renal tubule, are bright yellow, and resemble cancer in all histological respects. When they are small they are innocent. By convention, they are called

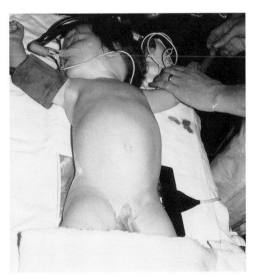

Figure 8.2 Wilms' tumour – a big lump in a wasted baby.

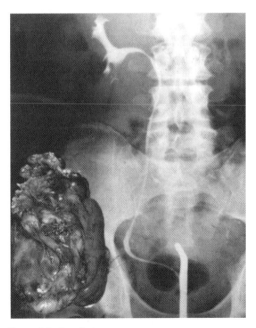

Figure 8.3 Grawitz tumour.

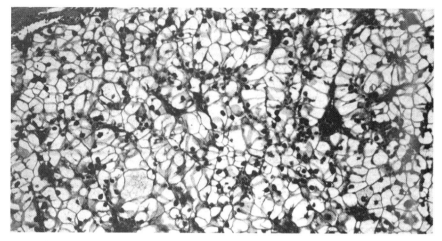

Figure 8.4 Typical clear-celled renal cell carcinoma of the kidney.

adenoma if they are less than 3 cm in diameter, and *cancer* if more than 3 cm. But metastases can occur from tumours which are less than 2 cm.

Grade

Typical clear-celled renal cell carcinoma of the kidney (Fig. 8.4) show a number of nuclear varied features which lead to a number of grading systems addressing this issue. Fuhrman's system has been most generally adopted. It is now recognised as an important independent prognostic factor. It is based on such features as nuclear size and shape and the presence or absence of prominent nuclei (Table 8.1).

Stage

The UICC system, based on the findings on CT scanning and pathological examination of the excised specimen is described in Fig. 8.5 and

Table 8.2. This allows stage grouping as seen in Table 8.3.

Clinical features

Today, most kidney cancers are detected *incidentally* when they are quite small because of an ultrasound scan done for some entirely unrelated reason. The classical symptoms of *haematuria, pain* and a *lump* are all features of late, large cancers (Fig. 8.6). Haematuria means that the cancer has already invaded the collecting system: pain means spread into the surrounding tissues a lump has to be very big indeed if it can be felt.

Neoplastic hormone syndromes

There is an interesting subgroup of patients present with features which can often be related to a specific chemical or hormone produced by the malignant renal cells Table 8.2.

Grade 1	Nuclear shape	Round, uniform
	Nucleoli	None
Grade 2	Nuclear shape	Slightly irregular
	Nucleoli	Visible at high power ×400 magnification
Grade 3	Nuclear shape	Very irregular outlines
	Nucleoli	Prominent visible at ×100 magnification
Grade 4	Nuclear shape	Bizzare and multilobed spindle-shaped cells
	Nucleoli	Prominent

Table 8.1 Fuhrman grading system.

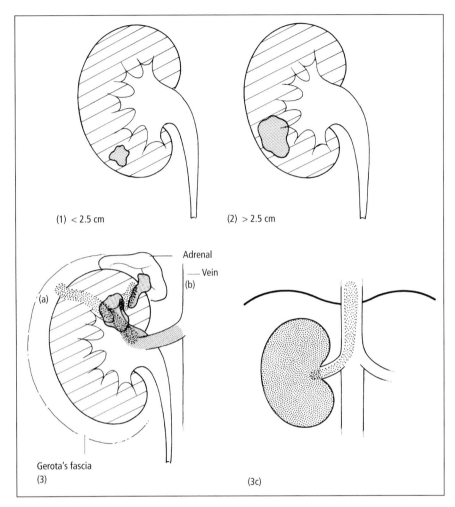

(1) < 2.5 cm

(2) > 2.5 cm

Adrenal

Vein

(b)

(a)

Gerota's fascia

(3)

(3c)

Figure 8.5 Stages of renal cell carcinoma.

Table 8.2 Neoplastic hormone syndromes in renal cell cancer.

Pyrogen	Loss of weight, pyrexia, night sweats, raised ESR
Erythropoietin	Erythrocytosis without increase in platelets
Marrow toxin	Anaemia
Renin	Hypertension
Parathyroid hormone	Hypercalcaemia
Stauffer's factor	Hepatosplenomegaly
Glucagon	Diarrhoea, enteropathy
Tumour proteins	Glomerulonephritis
Amyloid	Amyloid in contralateral kidney
Unknown factor	Paraneoplastic motoneurone disease

Table 8.3 International TNM system of staging for renal cell carcinoma (2002).

Pathological factor	Score
pT category of primary tumour	
pT1a	0
pT1b	2
pT2	3
pT3-4	4
Regional lymph node status	
pNx or pN0	0
pN1 or pN2	2
Tumour size	
<10 cm	0
>10 cm	1
Nuclear grade	
1 or 2	0
3 (= Fuhrman 3)	1
4 (= Fuhrman 4)	3
Histological tumour necrosis	
No	0
Yes	1

Table 8.4 Stage grouping.

Stage I	T1 N0 M0
Stage II	T2 N0 M0
Stage III	T3 N0 M0
	T1, T2, T3 N1 M0
Stage IV	T4 N0, N1 M0
	Any T N2 M0
	Any T Any N M1

are distinct in terms of the likelihood of malignancy (Table 8.4).

The intravenous urogram (IVU) and CT scan show a mass distorting the collecting system (Fig. 8.7) but may not be able to distinguish between a collection of cysts and cancer. With a very large tumour, one needs to know whether the vena cava has been invaded: here spiral magnetic resonance imaging (MRI) is more accurate than either CT or a cavogram (Fig. 8.8). Many tumours are detected only when a distant metastasis is biopsied and the unmistakable histological picture of a renal cell cancer is found.

Investigations

Ultrasound shows a mass in the kidney which contains echoes. Strict ultrasound criteria for simple cysts have been identified. Bosniak classification divides renal cystic lesions into four categories that

Treatment

Small tumours

Many tumours now detected incidentally in the course of ultrasound and CT scanning can be

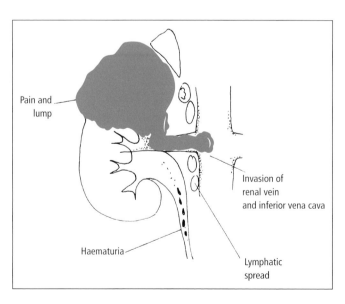

Pain and lump

Invasion of renal vein and inferior vena cava

Haematuria

Lymphatic spread

Figure 8.6 Clinical features of renal cell carcinoma.

Table 8.5 Bosniak renal cyst classification system.

Category	Wall	Septa	Calcification	Solid component	Measures water density	Enhance
I	Hairline thin	No	No	No	Yes – uniformly	No
II	Hairline thin	Few (<1 mm thick)	Yes – fine thickened	No	Yes	No
IIF*	Smooth thickening	Multiple	Yes – thick and nodular	No	Some parts may	No
III	Thickened or irregular	Yes (>1 mm thick)	Yes – thick and irregular	No	Some parts may	Yes
IV	Thickened or irregular	Yes	Yes	Yes	Some parts may	Yes

*These lesions are poorly defined but possess features requiring follow-up.

removed leaving a safe clear margin of healthy tissue by *partial nephrectomy*.

Partial nephrectomy

After exposing the kidney, the renal artery is secured. If it seems likely that the operation will be a

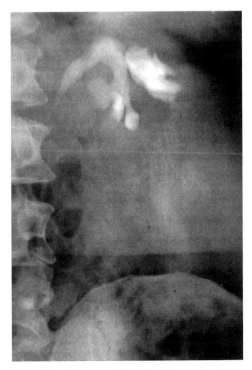

Figure 8.7 IVU showing left renal pelvis grossly distorted by huge soft tissue mass arising from the lower pole.

long one, the kidney is packed in sterile ice slush. The cancer is then removed with a clear margin (checked by frozen section). Every vessel is then suture ligated to secure complete haemostasis. In selected cases this operation can be done laparoscopically.

Large tumours

Radical nephrectomy

Through a generous incision (either vertical or transverse – according to the build of the patient (Fig. 8.9) – the colon and duodenum are reflected from the front of the kidney (Fig. 8.10). The renal artery is ligated. Then the vein is divided between ligatures, and an intact block of tissue is then removed containing the kidney, all the surrounding fat inside Gerota's fascia, and the lymph nodes along the side of the aorta (on the left) or the vena cava (on the right). When tumour is found growing into the renal vein, after taping the cava, lumbar veins and opposite renal veins, the vena cava is clamped and the lump of tumour removed cleanly (Fig. 8.11).

When preoperative investigations have shown that the tumour has extended along the inferior vena cava into the heart the abdominal incision is prolonged through the sternum. The patient is put on cardiac bypass. The vena cava is secured below and above the liver and the tumour extension removed. Worthwhile survival has been reported following this intervention.

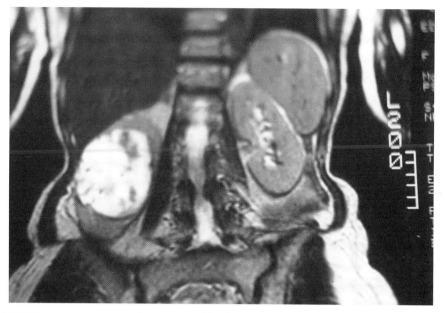

Figure 8.8 MRI image showing renal cell carcinoma in right kidney.

The choice between partial and total nephrectomy, either performed in an open fashion or laparoscopically, is an ongoing topic for debate. Patients with a solitary kidney, severe renal insufficiency or bilateral renal masses are candidates for partial nephrectomy if possible as more radical surgery would render them dependent on dialysis. Suitability for partial nephrectomy depends on the size and position of the tumour and the experience of the surgeon. The disadvantages of partial nephrectomy include tumour recurrence in the remaining part of the kidney and the potential complications and morbidity of the procedure. Frozen section pathological examination of the tumour margin seems to be unreliable and its routine use cannot be supported.

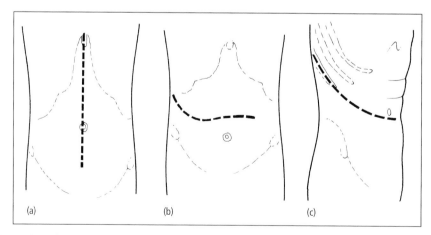

Figure 8.9 Incisions for radical nephrectomy chosen according to the site and size of the tumour and the build of the patient.

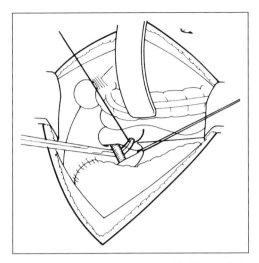

Figure 8.10 The renal artery is ligated before mobilising the mass.

Prognosis

If the cancer is confined to the kidney, nephrectomy alone is followed by over 80% 5-year survival. The outlook is worse when the lymph nodes are involved or the fat and vena cava are invaded. Sometimes, miraculously, distant metastases go away once the primary tumour has been removed, suggesting that there might be a powerful natural immune system against renal cell cancer although good survival is only seen in otherwise fit patients whose tumours are relatively well differentiated. Analysis of prognostic factors using the Leibovich scoring system has increased our predictive capability and nomograms are being developed for estimating the probability of survival after radical nephrectomy (see Tables 8.5 and 8.6). Chemotherapy based on inhibiting the factors involved tumour growth and angiogenesis have proved to be effective (Sunitinib, Sorafenib and RAD100 Everolimus are examples of a growing list).

Rare tumours that imitate renal cell cancer

B: Benign multilocular cysts imitate all the radiological, CT and ultrasonic features of the cystic form of a Grawitz cancer.

A: Angiomyolipoma is a tumour which is sometimes associated with *tuberose sclerosis*. Its

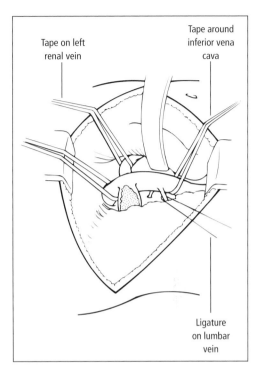

Figure 8.11 Extension of tumour into the inferior vena cava: the veins are all taped before opening the vena cava.

Table 8.6 Leibovich score.

Pathological factor	Score
pT category of primary tumour	
pT1a	0
pT 1b	2
pT2	3
pT3-4	4
Regional lymph node status	
pNx or pN0	0
pN1 or pN2	2
Tumour size	
<10 cm	0
>10 cm	1
Nuclear grade	
1 or 2	0
3 (= Fuhrman 3)	1
4 (= Furhman 4)	3
Histological tumour necrosis	
No	0
Yes	1

Group	Scores	Year 5 (%)	Year 10 (%)
Low risk	0–2	97.1	92.5
Intermediate risk	3–5	73.8	64.3
High risk	6 or more	31.2	23.6

Table 8.7 Estimated metastasis free survival.

content of fat gives it an unmistakable appearance in the CT scan. Some of these tumours bleed spontaneously and cause fatal retroperitoneal haemorrhage. Others become malignant, so they should always be removed.

Urothelial cancer of the renal pelvis and ureter

The renal pelvis and ureter are lined with urothelium which is identical with that of the bladder, and gives rise to identical urothelial or transitional cell cancer. Urothelial cancer is seen in patients with recurrent bladder cancers and in the West is associated with smoking, and all the causes of interstitial nephritis and papillary necrosis.

Pathology

Urothelial cancer in the *upper* tract, like that in the bladder, is classified in three grades: 1, 2 and 3. Metaplasia of the transitional epithelium gives rise to squamous cell cancers and adenocarcinomas, both of which are usually very anaplastic. The tumours spread directly into the muscle of the pelvis and the renal parenchyma as well as into the surrounding fat. They can seed further down the urinary tract and they metastasise via lymph nodes rather than veins.

Clinical features

Haematuria is the most important symptoms: pain is late.

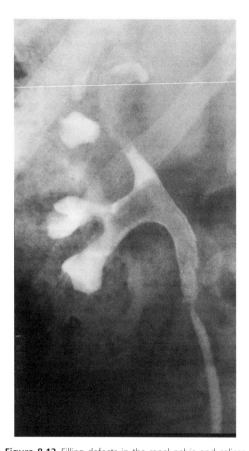

Figure 8.12 Filling defects in the renal pelvis and calices from multifocal urothelial carcinoma of the right kidney.

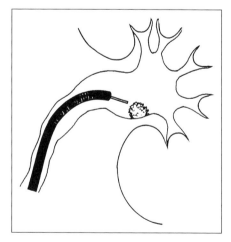

Figure 8.13 Coagulation of a small tumour in the renal pelvis with the YAG laser through a flexible ureteroscope.

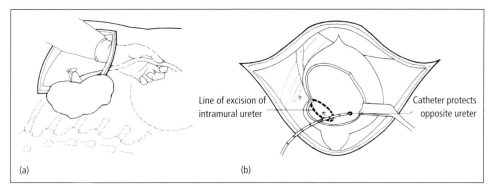

Line of excision of
intramural ureter

Catheter protects
opposite ureter

(a)

(b)

Figure 8.14 Nephroureterectomy: (a) the kidney and ureter are mobilised and (b) the lower end of the ureter is removed with a cuff of trigone.

Investigations

The IVU shows a filling defect (Fig. 8.12) which may be difficult to detect when the tumour is small. Malignant cells may be recognised on cytological examination of the urine in G2 and G3 tumours. The CT and ultrasound scans do not help. A retrograde ureterogram gives a clearer picture of the filling defect, and a small brush may be used to acquire cells from the tumour for cytology. Many of these tumours can now be visualised with a ureteroscope through which a biopsy can be obtained.

Treatment

The majority of these cancers are G3, multifocal, and have already invaded the muscle of the renal pelvis, so that the correct treatment is nephroureterectomy. However, when the tumour is *well differentiated* and still uninvasive, it is sometimes possible to perform a conservative resection. Some of the smaller tumours can be effectively

treated with a Holmium:YAG or Neodymium:YAG laser (Fig. 8.13).

Others are treated percutaneously. A working sheath is introduced as for percutaneous nephrolithotomy and the tumour is coagulated with a laser or diathermy. There is a risk that tumour cells may be implanted in the track so postoperative radiation is given. When local resection is not appropriate, the kidney may be approached through the 12th rib tip approach, as for pyelolithotomy the pelvis is opened, and the tumour locally excised.

Nephroureterectomy

The kidney and ureter are removed *en bloc* (Fig. 8.14) by either open surgery or laparoscopically. If the ureter is left behind there is an almost inevitable chance of recurrence. In G3 tumours, adjuvant radiotherapy is often given before the nephroureterectomy, or combination chemotherapy given afterwards.

Chapter 9

Vascular disorders of the kidney and hypertension

Arterial infarction

Since the branches of the renal artery do not anastomose with each other if one of them is blocked its territory becomes infarcted. This is sometimes seen with mural thrombi following cardiac infarction. The patient has loin pain and haematuria, and a urogram will show atrophy of a segment of the kidney. If the main renal artery is blocked the entire parenchyma atrophies, but the pelvis and collecting systems are not affected (Fig. 9.1).

Venous thrombosis

The veins of the kidney intercommunicate freely with each other and with the veins in the surrounding fat so that even when the main renal vein is completely blocked recovery is usually complete (Fig.9.2). Renal vein thrombosis is sometimes seen in children who are ill and dehydrated. They have pain and swelling in the loin, with profuse haematuria. A urogram may show no contrast on that side for a while, but in spite of this, recovery may be complete. In adults renal vein thrombosis may occur if intravenous contrast medium is given to a patient with amyloid.

Lecture Notes: Urology, 6th edition. By John Blandy and Amir Kaisary. Published 2009 by Blackwell Publishing. ISBN: 978-1-4051-2270-2.

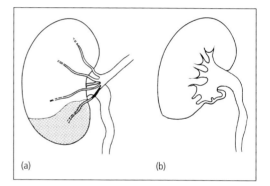

(a)   (b)

Figure 9.1 Embolism in a segmental artery leads to infarction and atrophy of an entire segment.

Aneurysm of the renal artery

Aneurysms of the renal artery may be saccular or fusiform, and may involve the main segmental branches as well as the main artery. The wall is often calcified (Fig. 9.3). On clinical examination a bruit may be heard over the kidney. The diagnosis depends on good selective angiography.

Treatment

The risk of spontaneous rupture in a saccular aneurysm increases with size. Those that are less than 1 cm in diameter can safely be kept under observation, but those more than 2 cm should be operated on. Fusiform aneurysms may be

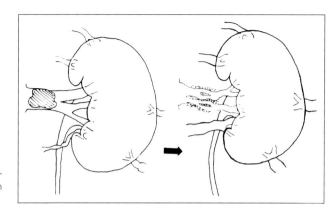

Figure 9.2 Blockage of renal vein is seldom followed by infarction due to the rich collateral venous circulation.

associated with patchy narrowing of branches of the renal artery causing hypertension, and may require reconstruction.

Arteriovenous aneurysms

Most of these follow trauma, including that of taking a renal biopsy. The shunting effect may give rise to heart failure. A similar kind of arteriovenous fistula is seen in some types of very vascular renal cell cancer. Nephrectomy is usually necessary but increasingly utilisation of

selective embolisation techniques can be successful in occluding the fistula and stops bleeding (Fig. 9.4).

Renal hypertension

The juxtaglomerular apparatus continually monitors the pressure in the glomerular arteriole (Fig. 9.5). When the pressure is lowered, it secretes *renin*, an enzyme which splits *angiotensinogen* – one of the alpha 2-globulins in serum – to release

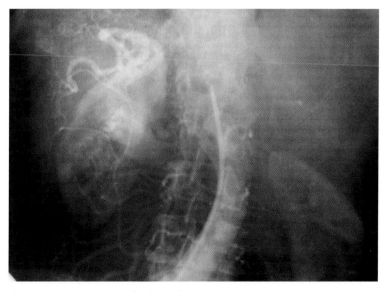

Figure 9.3 Arteriogram showing aneurysm of right renal artery.

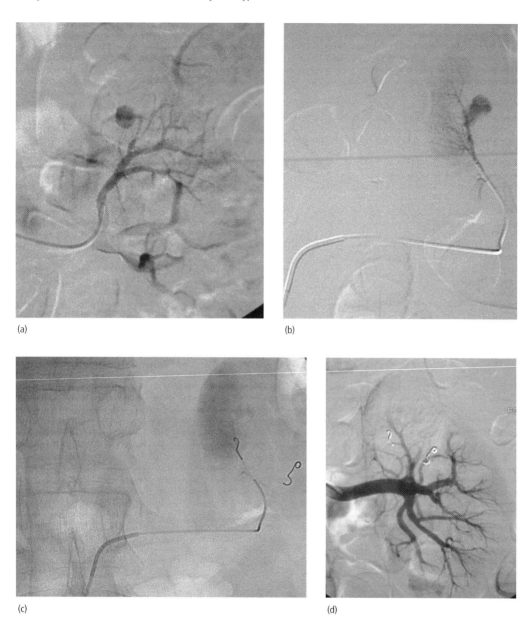

(a)

(b)

(c)

(d)

Figure 9.4 An arteriovenous post-traumatic fistula treated with embolisation.

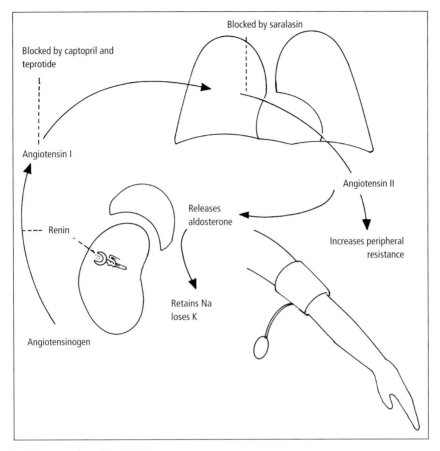

Figure 9.5 Mechanism of renal hypertension.

angiotensin I. This is at first inactive, but on passing through the lungs it is converted into *angiotensin II*, which has two powerful pharmacological effects that raise the blood pressure:

1 it constricts peripheral arteries; and
2 it stimulates the outer layer of the adrenal cortex to secrete *aldosterone* which makes the distal renal tubules conserve sodium and water and so increases the blood volume.

This renin–angiotensin mechanism can be triggered by a whole range of disorders of the kidney, including scarring from whatever cause, tuberculosis, cancer, polycystic disease, trauma and hydronephrosis. Its most striking form is seen when the main renal artery is stenosed.

Investigation

A renal cause should always be sought in a young patient with hypertension because it can usually be corrected. An intravenous urogram (IVU) will reveal hydronephrosis or scarring. Dimercaptosuccinic acid (DMSA) isotope studies show an impaired blood flow, and angiography with digital vascular imaging will localise the stenosis in the renal artery.

Although one can measure plasma renin, it is easier to detect its action indirectly. Captopril and teprotide block the release of angiotensin II in the lungs. Saralasin blocks the pharmacological effects of angiotensin II.

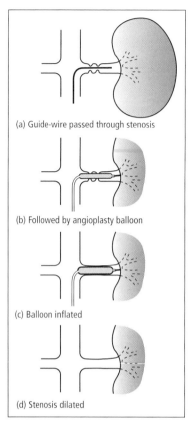

(a) Guide-wire passed through stenosis

(b) Followed by angioplasty balloon

(c) Balloon inflated

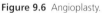

(d) Stenosis dilated

Figure 9.6 Angioplasty.

Patch on stenosed renal artery

By-pass graft from aorta to distal healthy renal artery

Figure 9.8 Patching or bypassing a renal artery stenosis.

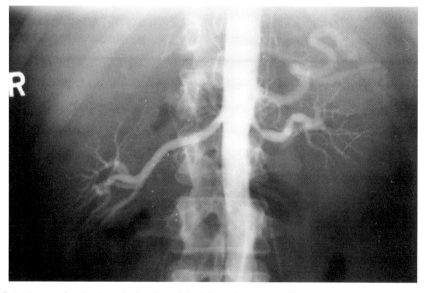

Figure 9.7 Angiogram showing irregular beading of the left renal artery from fibromuscular dysplasia.

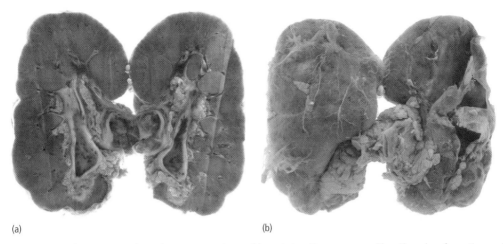

(a)   (b)

Figure 9.9 Renal artery stenosis nephrectomy specimen: (a) post-stenotic aneurysm with a thrombus formation and (b) multiple petechiae noted submucosally in the renal pelvis. Note the overall small size of the kidney.

If these substances lower the blood pressure, one can assume that renin is responsible.

Renal artery stenosis

There are two main causes of renal artery stenosis:
• Atheroma may form a plaque at the origin of the main renal artery which can be treated by dilatation with a balloon catheter – *angioplasty* (Fig. 9.6).
• In dysplasia the artery is irregularly narrowed like a string of beads (Fig. 9.7). This can be bypassed with a graft, or enlarged by adding on a patch (Fig. 9.8).

When there is a small scarred kidney, it is usually futile to try to deal with the narrowed artery, and better to perform nephrectomy. Arterial stenosis can occasionally lead to a post-stenotic aneurismal formation. A thrombus forming in a post-stenotic arterial aneurysm can be a source of emboli (see Fig. 9.9). When both kidneys are affected, one may obtain a useful improvement in renal function and avoid the need for dialysis by operating on the arteries.

Patients with significant renal artery disease could benefit from several revascularisation techniques. Aortorenal bypass with a free graft of autogenous blood vessels have been attempted (utilising the hypogastric artery or the saphenous vein). Percutaneous endoluminal balloon dilatation of arterial stenosis (angioplasty) gained interest which culminated in proceeding to stenting. The quality of the abdominal aorta and visceral arteries walls and atherosclerotic changes play a major role in patient case selection and possible outcome.

Chapter 10

The adrenal gland

Surgical anatomy

Each adrenal gland lies just medial to the upper pole of the kidney. The arteries supplying the
adrenals arise from the aorta, phrenic and renal
arteries and are all quite small. The right adrenal
vein drains into the vena cava: it is short and easily torn. The left adrenal vein enters the left renal
vein (Fig. 10.1).

The adrenal gland is like a three-layer sandwich –
the *cortex* – folded over a jam filling – the *medulla*.
The outer layer of the cortex – the *zona glomeru-
losa*, secretes aldosterone. The middle layer, the
zona fasciculata, secretes cortisol. The inner layer,
zona reticularis, secretes androgens (Fig. 10.2). The
medulla is made of sympathetic nerve endings and
pheochromocytes which secrete adrenaline and noradrenaline.

Adrenal tumours

Tumours can arise from any part of the adrenal,
and may or may not secrete the appropriate
hormone.

Non-functioning tumours

These are usually detected by accident in the
course of an ultrasound or computed tomography
(CT) scan. From time to time they present with
metastases. Size is the usual, but rather oversimple
guide to malignancy, i.e. tumours less than 3 cm
diameter are mostly benign, those more than 6 cm
diameter are usually malignant. Each case has to be
considered on its merits and sometimes a biopsy is
required.

Zona glomerulosa tumours (Conn's syndrome)

These may be single or multiple and may occur on
both sides. They are usually benign. The secretion
of aldosterone leads to retention of sodium causing hypertension, and loss of potassium causing
weakness. The diagnosis is made by the combination of hypertension, low plasma [K], high level of
aldosterone, and low level of renin. It is confirmed
by giving spironolactone which reverses the picture. The patient can often be controlled with
spironolactone but its side effects, e.g. enlargement of the breasts, indigestion and impotence,
may be unbearable and the patient may prefer an
operation. The adrenals are exposed through two
12th rib tip incisions. If a single adenoma is found
the entire adrenal is removed: if both adrenals
are involved with multiple adenomas, both are

Lecture Notes: Urology, 6th edition. By John Blandy and
Amir Kaisary. Published 2009 by Blackwell Publishing.
ISBN: 978-1-4051-2270-2.

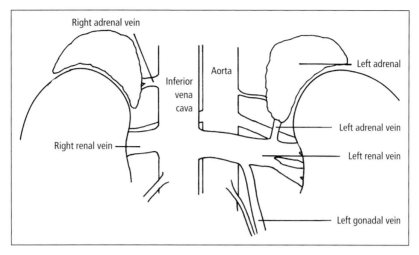

Figure 10.1 Anatomical relations of the adrenal gland.

removed and adrenal replacement given afterwards. Laparoscopy approach can be offered by experts in the technique.

Zona fasciculata tumours (Cushing's syndrome)

The excess of cortisol gives the patient a buffalo hump at the back of the neck, hirsutes, a red face, subcutaneous haemorrhages, cutaneous striae, hypertension, diabetes and osteoporosis which may lead to pathological fractures (Fig. 10.3).

There may be a single cortisol-secreting tumour, or there may be bilateral hyperplasia. In turn hyperplasia is sometimes caused by a basophil adenoma of the pituitary which is secreting adrenocorticotrophic hormone (ACTH). Very rarely the

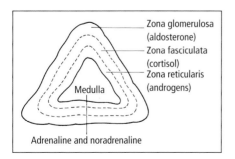

Figure 10.2 The folded sandwich arrangement of the adrenal.

ACTH may be secreted by another tumour, e.g. carcinoma of the bronchus.

The diagnosis of Cushing's syndrome is made by measuring the urinary metabolites of cortisol, the 17-hydroxycorticosteroids. If due to ACTH stimulation, an intravenous dose of ACTH will increase these: if there is a primary adrenal tumour, a dose of dexamethasone will lower them.

If a CT/MRI scan reveals a primary adrenal tumour it is removed. If there is hyperplasia of both adrenals, a pituitary tumour must be excluded, and if none is found, then both adrenals are removed and adrenal replacement given afterwards.

Zona reticulosa tumours (virilisation)

Isolated androgen-secreting tumours causing virilisation are rare but an excess of androgens is often secreted by malignant adrenal tumours that are also producing cortisol. In children this causes increased growth, hirsutes, enlarged genitalia, a deep voice and, in girls, precocious menstruation. In adults there may be acne, hirsutes and disturbance of menstruation.

Tumours of the adrenal medulla (pheochromocytoma)

Pheochromocytoma may occur in association with inherited disorders such as the multiple endocrine

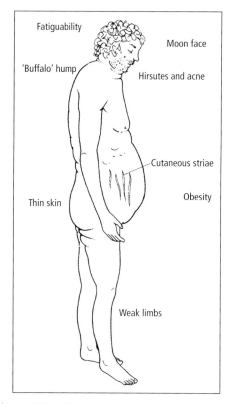

Figure 10.3 Cushing's syndrome.

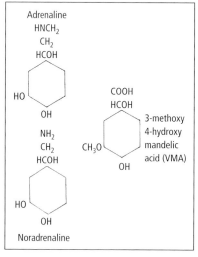

Figure 10.4 Adrenaline, noradrenaline and VMA.

neoplasia type II and von Hippel–Lindau disease. They arise either in the adrenal medulla or on the aorta at the origin of the inferior mesenteric artery, and very rarely, in the bladder. The excess of adrenaline and noradrenaline causes paroxysms of hypertension with headache, sweating, flushing, tremor and pain in the chest.

Diagnosis is based on a 24-hour collection of urine acidified with hydrochloric acid, and measured for adrenaline, noradrenaline, and their metabolic end product, vanillylmandelic acid (VMA) (Fig. 10.4). During this test the patient avoids anything containing vanilla, e.g. bananas, chocolate and coffee. Although these tumours are so vascular that they show up vividly in an angiogram, but are more easily located with a CT scan or MRI.

The tumour must be removed. About 10% are malignant. To protect the patient from a sudden surge of catecholamines, phenoxybenzamine is given to block the alpha-receptors and propanolol to block the beta-receptors. Even though these have been blocked, the tumour is handled as little as possible until the veins have all been ligated, at which moment the anaesthetist must be ready to deal with a fall in blood pressure. How the tumour is approached depends on its position: tumours near the adrenal are reached through a 12th rib tip incision; those near the inferior mesenteric artery through a midline laparotomy.

Neuroblastoma

These are malignant tumours arising from nerve cell elements. They occur in toddlers, frequently with widespread metastases. The most common site of origin of the primary is in the region of the adrenal, but they can arise anywhere. They grow to an enormous size, and displace the kidney downwards. They must be distinguished from Wilms' tumours. Occasionally, they secrete catecholamines and elevated levels of VMA are found in the urine. They are treated in specialised children's hospitals by a combination of surgery and chemotherapy.

Chapter 11

Renal failure

Acute or chronic renal failure? It is sometimes not easy to differentiate between these two conditions. The history, duration of symptoms and measurements of renal function may help make the distinction. A rapid change of serum urea and creatinine suggests an acute process; whereas presence of a normochromic and normocytic anaemia suggests chronic disease. A renal ultrasound scan may help: small, shrunken kidneys seen on ultrasound scan usually indicate chronic renal failure.

Acute renal failure

In acute renal failure, there is an abrupt deterioration of renal function which is usually reversible over a period of days or weeks. The causes of acute renal failure are categorised into three groups: (1) pre-renal; (2) interstitial or renal parenchymal; and (3) post-renal or obstructive. The causes may occur in combination (Fig. 11.1).

1 Pre-renal failure is usually caused by inadequate renal perfusion because of hypovolaemia, hypotension, impaired cardiac function or renal vascular disease. The end result is renal ischaemia and subsequently oliguria.

2 Interstitial or renal parenchymal disease can be caused by conditions such as acute tubular necro-

Lecture Notes: Urology, 6th edition. By John Blandy and Amir Kaisary. Published 2009 by Blackwell Publishing. ISBN: 978-1-4051-2270-2.

sis, vasculitis, acute tubulointerstitial nephritis, haemolytic uraemic syndrome, pre-eclampsia and thrombotic thrombocytopaenic purpura.

3 Post-renal or obstructive causes of acute renal failure result from obstruction of the urinary tract at any point from the renal calices to the urethra, e.g. stones in the kidney or ureter, transitional cell carcinomas, bladder outlet obstruction from enlarged prostate or urethral stricture and iatrogenic causes such as blocked urinary catheters and accidental ligation of ureters during surgery.

Pathology

In acute renal failure the kidney is swollen. The blood is usually shunted from cortex to medulla so that the medulla is congested and the cortex pale. Debris clogs up the tubules and resembles necrosis – hence the old term *acute tubular necrosis* – which is misleading because the condition is often reversible, especially when mainly caused by underperfusion. If the cause cannot be reversed, then the cortex does indeed die, and a line of calcification may appear at the edge of the dead tissue (Fig. 11.2).

Clinical features and management

The cause of the acute renal failure will have its own particular symptoms, e.g. septicaemia or multiple trauma. Against this background three phases

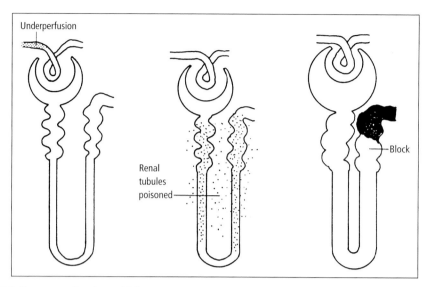

Figure 11.1 The causes of acute renal failure.

can be distinguished: prodromal, oliguria–anuria and recovery.

• *Prodromal phase:* At first, while there is still some glomerular filtration, urine continues to form but is loaded with debris and granular casts.

• *Anuria or oliguria:* Next comes a stage when there may be either no urine at all, or too little to cope with the products of protein catabolism, e.g. urea, creatinine, potassium and phosphates. The blood urea, creatinine and potassium continue to rise, at a rate which is accelerated when there

is massive breakdown of tissue from trauma or sepsis.

• *Recovery:* At first the glomerular filtrate that starts to emerge is almost unprocessed by the sick tubules and is pale and isotonic. Soon the trickle is followed by such a huge volume of dilute urine that the patient may need many litres of fluid to prevent dehydration and keep up with the massive losses of water and sodium.

In pre-renal acute renal failure, patients usually complain of thirst or dizziness, with or without

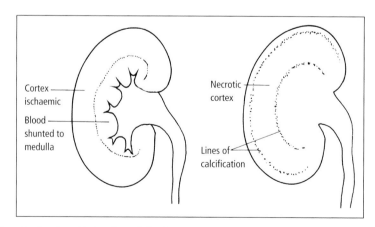

Figure 11.2 Necrosis of cortex with tramline calcification.

orthostatic hypotension. Weight loss occurs over days which reflects the degree of dehydration. Physical examination reveals signs of dehydration and also postural changes in blood pressure and pulse. The output of urine and central venous pressure are low, consistent with hypovolaemia. An increase in urine output in response to fluid challenge is usually diagnostic. The management of pre-renal acute renal failure involves calculated fluid replacement during which a central venous pressure line may be useful to ensure that the patient is not being overloaded with fluid.

When interstitial or renal parenchymal disease is causing the acute renal failure, there may be a history of sore throat (*Streptococcal glomerulonephritis*), upper respiratory tract infection, diarrhoea, recent use of antibiotics or recreational drugs. Patients may complain of bilateral loin pain, there may be frank haematuria, associated systemic sepsis and dehydration. Urine microscopy may reveal numerous red blood cells and leucocytes, together with cellular and granular casts. Thrombocytopaenia may be present on examination of the blood film and a renal biopsy will show the characteristics changes of glomerulonephritis. The management involves treating the cause of the renal failure, e.g. antibiotics for infection, removal of toxic drugs and suppression of immune mechanisms. Dialysis may be required.

In post-renal or obstructive causes of acute renal failure, the patient may complain of unilateral tenderness in the loin or renal angle. An example would be a stone causing unilateral ureteric obstruction and pain. There may not be a decrease in urine volume as there is usually a normal kidney on the other side. Indeed, large volumes of urine may be obtained from urethral catheterisation, particularly if the cause of the obstruction is in the lower urinary tract (e.g. benign prostatic hyperplasia or urethral stricture). A plain X-ray of the kidneys, ureters and bladder (KUB X-ray) may show a stone in the renal pelvis or ureter. An ultrasound scan may reveal a dilated renal pelvis and an intravenous urogram may show delayed excretion of contrast on the affected side. The treatment is to remove the cause of the obstruction, e.g. stenting for a ureteric calculus, transurethral resection of prostate or optical urethrotomy for urethral strictures.

Chronic renal failure

Chronic renal failure is the presence of longstanding and usually progressive impairment in renal function. The many causes of chronic renal failure are classified according to the general aetiology of the disease:
1 congenital causes such as adult or infantile polycystic kidney disease;
2 glomerular disease such as systemic lupus erythematosus, Wegener's granulomatosis and amyloidosis;
3 vascular diseases such as atherosclerosis and vasculitis;
4 tubulointerstitial diseases caused by drug overdose, tuberculosis and nephrocalcinosis; and
5 urinary tract obstruction caused by, for example, benign prostatic hyperplasia.

Clinical features and management

There are many clinical features of chronic renal failure listed below:
• Generalised malaise, nausea, loss of libido and forgetfulness.
• Hypertension and signs of volume or fluid overload.
• Retarded and stunted growth in children.
• Skin: itching, pigmentation and jaundice.
• Anaemia: want of erythropoietin leads to anaemia. Synthetic erythropoietin can correct this distressing feature.
• Neuropathy from loss of myelin in peripheral nerves causes weakness, numbness and paraesthesiae, notably in the feet.
• Pericarditis may result in a pericardial effusion; it is a warning that the patient is being underdialysed.
• Osteomalacia as the bowel becomes less sensitive to vitamin D, and so less calcium is absorbed. Growing bone is imperfectly calcified, forming

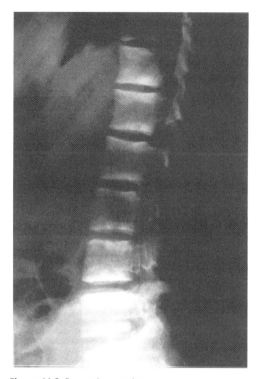

Figure 11.3 Rugger-jersey spine.

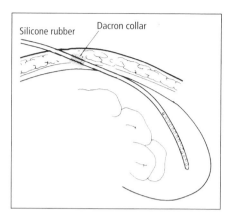

Figure 11.4 Peritoneal dialysis with Tenckhoff cannula.

Dialysis

Peritoneal dialysis

A silicone catheter is placed permanently in the pelvis (Fig. 11.4) and dialysis fluid is run in, left for several hours, and run out again after creatinine and products of catabolism have diffused into the fluid. Patients perform the instillation themselves. There are three main forms of peritoneal dialysis:

1 Continuous ambulatory peritoneal dialysis is the most common. Up to 3 L of dialysate are allowed to run into the peritoneal cavity, run out, and replaced three to five times a day.

2 Nightly intermittent peritoneal dialysis using an automated device which performs the fluid exchanges whilst the patient is asleep.

3 Tidal dialysis allows the residual volume within the peritoneal cavity to be continuously cycled and exchanged with a smaller volume of dialysate.

Complications from peritoneal dialysis are due to infection. Peritonitis may be caused by an infected catheter or dialysate fluid. Minimal handling of the catheter and strict aseptic techniques are taught to all patients for self-administering peritoneal dialysis.

osteoid rather than true bone – *osteomalacia* – which is weak and prone to fracture. At the same time phosphate accumulates and lowers the plasma [Ca], which stimulates the parathyroid to secrete more parathyroid hormone (see Fig. 7.7). In turn more calcium is leached from the bones and deposited in soft tissues as heterotopic calcification which can cause stiffness of joints, especially in the middle ear, leading to *deafness*, as well as the *rugger-jersey spine* where stripes of decalcified bone alternate with bands of soft tissue calcification (Fig. 11.3).

The management of chronic renal failure is at first conservative with restriction of dietary protein, potassium and phosphorus whilst taking care to maintain sodium balance. The patient is weighed every day. If conservative measures fail to control the progress of chronic renal failure, then dialysis may have to be needed.

Haemodialysis

Blood from the patient is allowed to flow over a semi-permeable membrane separating it from

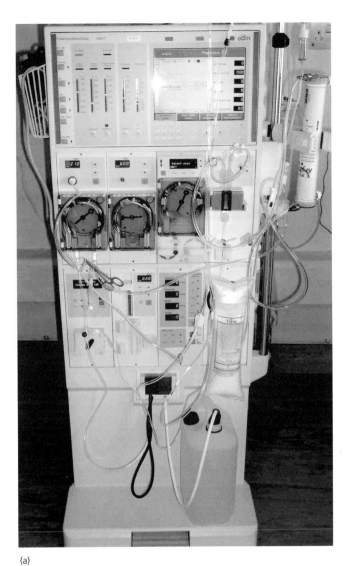

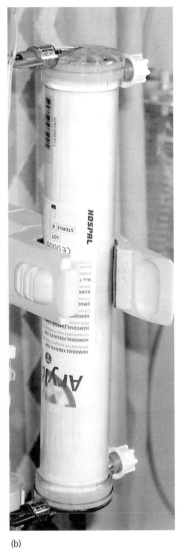

(a)   (b)

Figure 11.5 (a) Artificial kidney and (b) disposable cartridge.

dialysis fluid. There are a variety of devices, some of which are disposable and others used several times (Fig. 11.5). Unwanted products of catabolism diffuse out of the blood, while protein and red cells are retained. Access to the bloodstream is provided by an arteriovenous fistula, vascular grafts, subclavian perm-catheters or a *Scribner shunt* (Fig. 11.6) tied into a paired artery and vein. All these methods provide rapid and repetitive access into the vascular system. For pro-longed dialysis, a peripheral artery is anastomosed to a vein to form an arteriovenous fistula. Within a few weeks large varicose veins have formed into which the patient inserts needles enabling blood to run out through the machine and back again (Fig. 11.7). Repeated needling eventually leads to thrombosis or infection of these fistulae and every year more ingenious techniques are devised to provide suitable *vascular access* for intermittent haemodialysis.

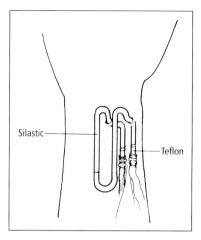

Figure 11.6 Scribner shunt.

Renal transplantation

The operation is in principle quite simple. A kidney from a living related donor or a cadaver is placed in one or other iliac fossa. The renal artery is anastomosed to the internal or external iliac artery, and the renal vein to the external iliac vein. The ureter is led through a tunnel into the bladder to prevent reflux (Fig. 11.8).

Obtaining cadaver kidneys

It is always a waste when kidneys that could save two lives are allowed to decay in a dead patient.

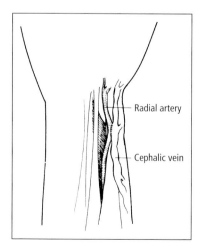

Figure 11.7 Cimino fistula.

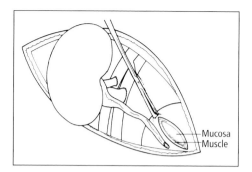

Figure 11.8 Renal transplant in right iliac fossa: the ureter is placed in a submucosal tunnel to prevent reflux.

Relatives seldom refuse to give permission for kidneys to be used, and then usually for religious reasons. The shortage of donors does not stem from the refusal of relatives, but from failure on the part of doctors and nurses to ask for permission, and a shortage of staff and facilities in intensive care units to keep patients on a ventilator after they are clearly brain-dead.

The donor

Suitable donors must not have infection or cancer (except for some brain tumours). They should have extensive and irrecoverable brain damage, e.g. from severe head injury, intracranial haemorrhage, cardiac arrest or respiratory arrest. Such patients must be maintained on a ventilator. Strict tests are carried out to make sure that the brain damage is irreversible. Since not only kidneys but also other organs such as the heart, lungs and liver might be usable, the opportunity should never be lost to consider the possibility of using more than one organ.

The major histocompatibility system

There is a strong positive correlation between histocompatibility matching for the human lymphocyte antigens (HLAs) (A, B and DR) and the success rate of transplant kidney survival. The transplant antigens, i.e. HLAs, are inherited on the sixth chromosome and expressed on the surface of every cell. Some are detected with serum antibodies (serum detected). Others can only be detected in mixed lymphocyte culture where the host lymphocytes react to foreign lymphocytes by swelling up and undergoing division (lymphocyte-activating determinants).

Rejection can only be prevented by getting an exact match between the HLA of host and donor but can be overcome by drugs which paralyse various components of the immune system. Immunosuppressive agents that are in common use at present include cyclosporin A, prednisolone, azathioprine, tacrolimus (FK506), rapamycin and mycophenolate mofetil:
• *Cyclosporin A* works by preventing the formation of cytotoxic T-cells by the host.
• *Prednisolone* seems to complement azathioprine and may affect the function of lymphocytes.
• *Azathioprine* works in a similar way, but is more toxic.
• *Tacrolimus (FK506)* works by suppressing interleukin-2 (IL-2) production from CD4 lymphocytes, and thus suppresses transplant rejection.
• *Rapamycin* similarly blocks the effect of IL-2.
• *Mycophenolate mofetil* is an anti-metabolite that inhibits purine synthesis and suppresses lymphocyte activity.

The prevention, recognition and treatment of rejection call for great skill and judgement.

HLA matching

Because of the way homologous pairs of chromosomes are split at meiosis and transmitted by haploid gametes from parents to children, each child receives half its genetic programming from one parent and half from the other (Fig. 11.9).

Living related donors

Transplants between siblings and between parents and children always share one complete set of transplant antigens, and generally do well. In a family with more than five children, one pair of siblings will always be identical with respect to their transplant antigens and if they exchange kidneys one might expect virtually no rejection. In fact there are other, weaker antigens, and

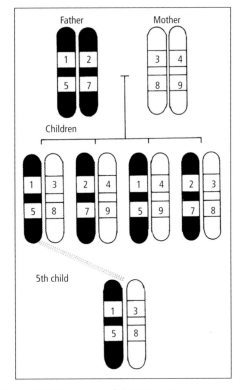

Figure 11.9 Inheritance of the HLA genes.

immunosuppressive drugs are needed except with identical twins. A good HLA match can double the survival of transplants and for this reason kidneys are moved from one centre to another to ensure the optimum match.

Living unrelated donors

The chance of finding a good HLA match in a living unrelated donor is always much smaller than in a relation, so much so that this is seldom done in the West, and is regarded as unethical and indeed unlawful if done as a commercial transaction.

Rejection episodes
Hyperacute rejection

Hyperacute rejection is similar to a blood transfusion reaction. A recipient may unwittingly have been sensitised to antigens on the donor kidney so that as soon as blood enters the kidney there is an accelerated second set reaction: within minutes the kidney becomes thrombosed. It is a humoral response mediated by recipient antibodies against the HLAs expressed on the donor renal vascular endothelium. For this reason, these pre-existing *cytotoxic antibodies* can be detected by a cross-match, which is always performed prior to any transplant.

Accelerated rejection

This is a *second set reaction* and begins within two or three days of the transplant: it can respond to prompt diagnosis and intensive immunosuppressive treatment.

Acute rejection

Acute rejection episodes are quite common, with approximately 40% of patients having at least one episode of acute rejection after renal transplantation. Episodes of rejection may occur at any time after the transplant, but are most common in the first few weeks. The kidney becomes tender and swollen. The patient is pyrexial and has pain over the transplant. The urine output diminishes, the diethylene triamine pentacetic acid clearance falls off (see p. 32) and Doppler studies show a diminished circulation. Fine-needle aspiration cytology from the graft shows blast cells and macrophages to be present, although T-lymphocytes are the predominant cells involved in this process. T-lymphocytes are stimulated and activated by foreign HLA antigens found in the transplanted kidney. Subsequently, IL-2 production by the recipient stimulates a cytotoxic T-cell response that promotes destruction of the graft.

Larger doses of immunosuppressive agents, especially cyclosporin A, usually reverse the reaction. Acute rejection may come on many months after a transplant and may be precipitated by failure to take immunosuppressive medication or a blood transfusion.

Chronic rejection

Chronic rejection is the process of gradual, progressive decrease in renal function. The gradual deterioration does not respond to immunosuppressive therapy and its underlying mechanisms are poorly understood. Eventually the transplanted kidney fails and must be removed. The patient returns to dialysis and may be put on the waiting list for another renal transplant.

Preservation of kidneys for transplantation

An ice-cold solution – the Wisconsin University solution – which imitates the content of intracellular fluid, is used to wash out the donor kidney, which is placed in a pair of sterile plastic bags in a container surrounded by ice. Such a kidney will recover normal function even after 36 hours of cold ischaemia time. What damages the kidney is the warm ischaemia time, i.e. the delay between cessation of perfusion of the kidney and its being cooled with preservative solution.

Long-term results of transplantation

There is a continuing and steady improvement in the results of renal transplantation. The current survival of renal transplants in the best transplant centres at the end of three years is more than 80% for living related and unrelated donors and approximately 76% for cadaveric renal transplants.

Chapter 12

The renal pelvis and ureter

Anatomy

The ureters descend in front of the psoas muscle and the iliohypogastric and ileoinguinal nerves. Halfway down, they are crossed in front by the vessels of the testis or ovary, and near the lower end by branches of the internal iliac artery and veins going to and from the uterus and bladder.

In women, the ureter is vulnerable during the operation of hysterectomy where it passes under the uterine artery and veins (Fig. 12.1). If there is bleeding, the ureter is easily injured in the course of efforts to secure haemostasis.

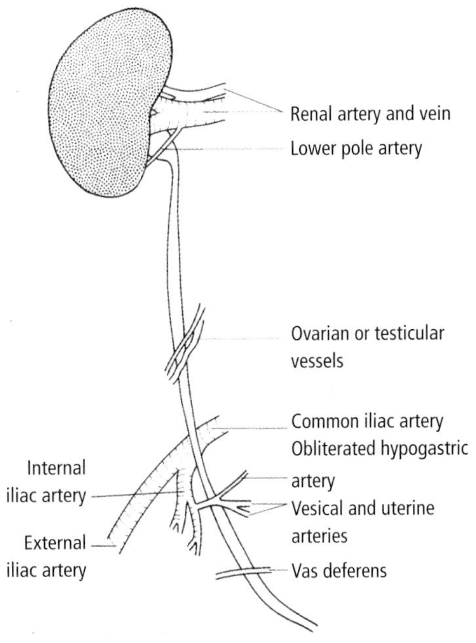

Blood supply

The main blood supply of the ureter comes down from the inferior segmental artery of the kidney (Fig. 12.2), which runs down the ureter, and is reinforced by unimportant small branches from the lumbar arteries. Towards the lower end, it is joined by an ascending branch of the superior vesical artery. If the ureter is divided near the bladder, this ascending branch is cut and the lower end of the ureter may be ischaemic.

Lecture Notes: Urology, 6th edition. By John Blandy and Amir Kaisary. Published 2009 by Blackwell Publishing. ISBN: 978-1-4051-2270-2.

Figure 12.1 Anatomical relations of the right ureter.

Nerve supply

Sensory nerves from the ureter follow a segmental pattern: the upper part, like the kidney, is supplied by T10, and pain is referred to the umbilicus. Lower down pain is referred to more caudal segments (L2,3,4) until pain from the lowest part of

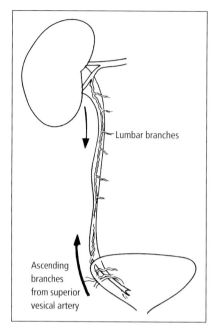

Figure 12.2 Blood supply of the ureter.

the ureter may be referred to the vulva or tip of the penis (S2,3) (Fig. 12.3).

Peristalsis

The ureter is lined by urothelium on a thin layer of submucosa (Fig. 12.4) outside of which the smooth muscle cells are connected with each other so that excitation passes along the muscle without the need for nerves or ganglia (Fig. 12.5). Peristalsis in the ureter can be provoked by pinching or irritation. As a result, the denervated ureter of a transplant functions perfectly well.

Ureteric peristaltic waves speed up as more urine is formed until the point is reached when the walls of the ureter no longer come together and it now functions as a drainpipe. To allow free movement of the ureter during peristalsis, it is surrounded by a thin slippery sheath of connective tissue.

Congenital abnormalities

The embryology of the ureter and some of the more important congenital abnormalities are de-

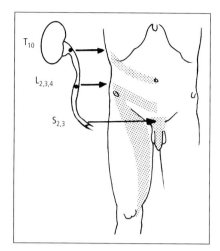

Figure 12.3 Pain from a stone in the ureter is referred to relevant dermatome.

scribed in Chapter 4. It may be helpful to be reminded of a few of them:

• In *duplex*, the ureteric bud branches early. The ureter from the smaller upper half of the kidney drains into the trigone caudal to that from the lower, larger half of the kidney.

• In *ectopic ureter*, the ureter from the upper half of the kidney opens into the vagina downstream of the urethral sphincter and causes continual incontinence (Fig. 12.6).

• In *ureterocele*, there is a balloon-like swelling where the ureter opens into the bladder, which may obstruct the ureter, allow a stone to form in

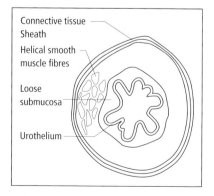

Figure 12.4 Transverse section of the ureter.

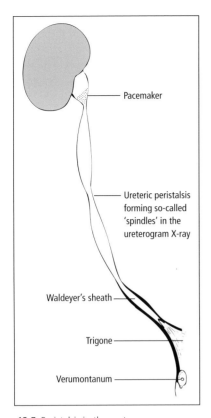

Figure 12.5 Peristalsis in the ureter.

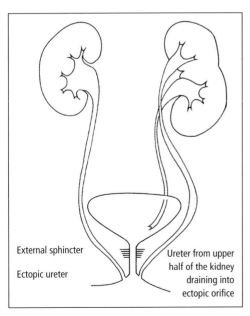

Figure 12.6 If an ectopic duplex ureter opens downstream of the sphincter there is incontinence.

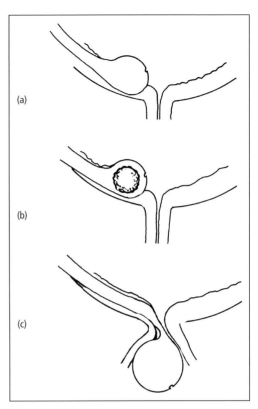

Figure 12.7 Ureteroceles may (a) cause no trouble at all; (b) cause obstruction and possibly a stone; (c) prolapse into the urethra to cause acute retention of urine.

its stagnant pool, or prolapse and obstruct the ure-thra. Most ureteroceles cause no trouble and need no treatment: the very large ones can be incised, but then there may be reflux requiring reimplantation (Fig. 12.7).

• *Reflux* has been considered in relation to urinary infection (Fig. 12.8). One of the less common conditions seen with duplex kidney is *yo-yo* reflux where urine runs from the lower half of the kidney to the upper one.

• One of the ureteric buds may fail to rendezvous with its part of the metanephros and no kidney is induced. The resulting *ureteric diverticulum* may harbour infection but usually needs no treatment at all.

• Ureteric *atresia* has been noted in connection with dysplasia and congenital cysts of the kidney.

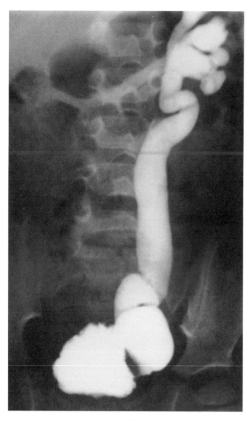

Figure 12.8 Vesicoureteric reflux.

Inflammation of the ureter

Acute

Acute ureteritis may explain much of the pain in the groin which patients so often describe during acute urinary infection. It is rarely investigated or documented, and always recovers completely with time and antibiotics.

Chronic

Non-specific

Ureteritis cystica
Following a prolonged urinary infection, the intravenous urogram (IVU) or ureterogram may show multiple rounded filling defects in the ureter and renal pelvis. These are caused by a particular

kind of chronic inflammation of the urothelium – ureteritis cystica – where little nests of urothelium get buried and swell up to form tiny cysts. It resolves completely when the underlying infection has been cured.

Specific

Tuberculosis
The ureter is often involved in tuberculosis.

Bilharziasis
The wall of the ureter is always involved in bilharziasis. Pairs of *Schistosoma* flukes nest in the submucosal veins and lay eggs which provoke chronic inflammation, turning the ureter into a stiff, inert tube which is dilated, obstructed and often calcified.

Diagnosis of obstruction in the ureter

To distinguish between a ureter that is obstructed from one that is widened from some other reason, renography is usually sufficient. Retrograde and antegrade radiological studies are usually provide the answer. Renal isotope studies, ^{99m}Tc benzoylmercaptoacetyltriglycerine (MAG3), ^{99m}Tc diethylenetriamine pentaacetic acid (DTPA) and ^{99m}Tc 2,3-dimercaptosuccinic acid (DMSA) are utilised to evaluate the renal function and impact of obstruction. In exceptional cases, Whitaker's test can be performed. A fine percutaneous nephrostomy tube is introduced into the renal pelvis and contrast medium is run in at a rate known to be greater than the maximum likely to be encountered during diuresis, e.g. 10 mL/min. If the pressure rises, it means there must be obstruction downstream in the ureter (Fig. 12.9).

Megaureter

This is a common and important entity in children. It causes confusion because it is often

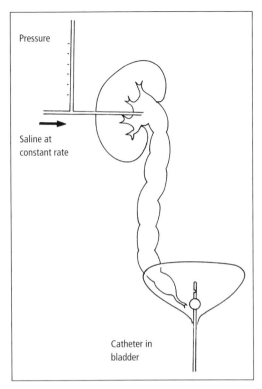

Figure 12.9 Whitaker's test.

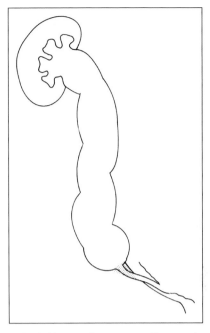

Figure 12.10 Obstructed ureter caused by stenosis at the lower end.

assumed that whenever a dilated ureter is discovered, there must necessarily be obstruction.
- *Reflux:* Most megaureters are caused by reflux.
- *Congenital stenosis* at the lower end of the ureter: A narrowing, from an unknown cause, occurs at the lower end of the ureter, giving rise to obstruction upstream (Fig. 12.10). Diagnosis may need a Whitaker's test.
- *Idiopathic:* In a number of boys the ureters are found to be huge, but there is no reflux, and no narrowing at the lower end. The cause is a mystery. One plausible suggestion is that at some time in foetal life there was a posterior urethral valve, which gave rise to gross obstruction and dilatation of the ureters, and then the valve ruptured spontaneously, leaving the child with large ureters without any apparent reason for them.
- *Diabetes insipidus:* Children may be unable to concentrate their urine, and a constant diuresis may be associated with dilated ureter.

Ureteric obstruction

Pelviureteric junction obstruction

This is a common condition. There is a ring of fibrous tissue where the renal pelvis joins the ureter of unknown cause. The renal pelvis and calices are obstructed and undergo dilatation – hydronephrosis (Fig. 12.11).

In the foetus, hydronephrosis is often detected by ultrasound scanning. Many of these show spontaneous cure during follow-up and surgical correction is only required if there is a deterioration in renal function, as judged by serial renography using DMSA.

In later life, hydronephrosis may be noted at any time. At first, its symptoms are often intermittent, so that pain occurs only when patients drink a lot, and because the pain follows a meal it is easy to misdiagnose a peptic ulcer.

The dilated renal pelvis bulges forwards between the two lower branches of the renal artery giving rise to the idea that an 'anomalous' renal artery is the cause of the obstruction (Fig. 12.12).

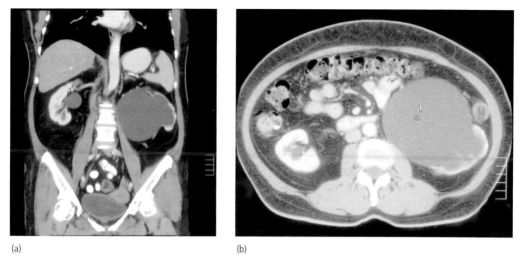

(a)   (b)

Figure 12.11 Hydronephrosis from obstruction at the pelviureteric junction: (a) longitudinal and (b) transverse.

Diagnosis

The difficulty in practice is to distinguish between a large baggy renal pelvis and one that is dilated because of obstruction. A DTPA renogram is performed, and after a few minutes frusemide is given to cause a diuresis. If there is obstruction, the isotope continues to accumulate in the renal pelvis: in a normal pelvis the isotope is washed away in the next few minutes (Fig. 12.13).

When the kidney is very distended, it is sometimes difficult to know whether it is worth trying to save it. A DMSA scan will show how much useful renal parenchyma is.

Management

Patients found by chance to have a large renal pelvis, but no DTPA evidence of obstruction, can safely be kept under observation year after

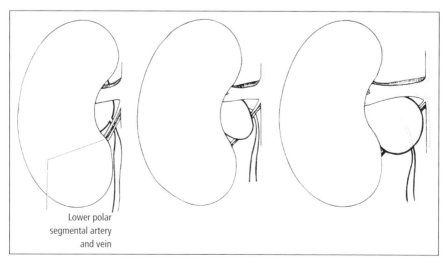

Lower polar
segmental artery
and vein

Figure 12.12 The obstructed renal pelvis often bulges out between the two lower segmental arteries.

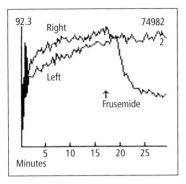

Figure 12.13 DTPA renogram showing retention of iso-tope in the left kidney in spite of frusemide.

year. In those with obvious obstruction, or severe symptoms, then something needs to be done to overcome the obstruction. There are several alternative methods:

• *Balloon dilatation:* An angioplasty catheter is passed up the ureter over a guidewire into the narrow segment and distended there. A double-J stent is left in situ for 10–14 days (Fig. 12.14).

• *Percutaneous ureterolysis:* A working sheath is introduced into the renal pelvis as for percutaneous nephrolithotomy (see Fig. 7.12). Using a nephroscope, a guidewire is passed down the ureter over which a knife is passed to incise the fibrous ring in the wall of the ureter. This is followed with a

double-J stent which is left in position for about 6 weeks (Fig. 12.15).

• *Pyeloplasty:* If these simple non-invasive methods are not feasible, or have been tried without success, a formal pyeloplasty is performed. Ureterogram is first made to define the length of the narrow segment of the ureter. Then the kidney is approached through an anterior transverse incision or laparoscopically. The peritoneum is reflected to reveal the pelvis and ureter. There are mainly two principles: dismembered and flap pyeloplasty techniques as shown in Fig. 12.16. The anastomosis is stented with a double-J stent for about 10 days. The follow-up is done with renography.

Retrocaval ureter

Very rarely the postcardinal veins of the embryo fail to become obliterated, and the ureter has to wind round behind the inferior vena cava. The IVU appearance is unmistakable (Fig. 12.17). There is no need to meddle with the little bit of ureter behind the vena cava. The lower end is detached and anastomosed to the dilated upper part just as in any other hydronephrosis.

Retroperitoneal fibrosis

Metastatic cancer, usually arising from the colon, may convert the retroperitoneal tissue into a hard plaque inside which the ureters cannot wriggle freely. Something similar is rarely seen in association with inflammation of the bowel in Crohn's disease or ulcerative colitis. But the most interesting of these types has no known cause, and is therefore called *idiopathic retroperitoneal fibrosis*.

These patients have backache, fever, weight loss, an elevated sedimentation rate and hypertension. The ureter is encased in a stiff plaque of fibrous tissue, and cannot writhe sideways or up and down, and so becomes obstructed, even though it is easy to pass a catheter up and down. By the time the diagnosis is made the patient is often severely uraemic. The same plaque of fibrous tissue encases the vena cava and aorta, and may extend up into the porta hepatis and mediastinum (Fig. 12.18).

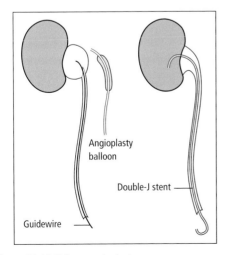

Figure 12.14 Balloon pyeloplasty.

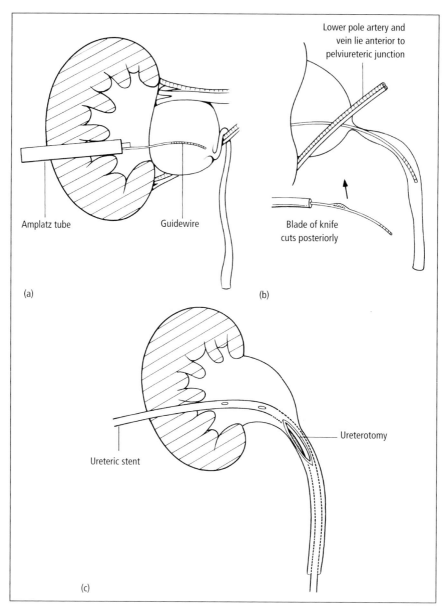

Figure 12.15 Percutaneous pyelolysis.

The first step is to relieve the obstruction with percutaneous nephrostomy. Once the patient has recovered from the uraemia, it is necessary to distinguish this from the other types of fibrosis listed above. Prednisolone has occasionally been reported to produce rapid and complete resolution of the obstruction, but more often the im-provement is slow and incomplete. A more certain method is to free the ureters from the surrounding fibrous tissue, and wrap them in omentum to stop it coming back (Fig. 12.19).

All these patients must be very carefully fol-lowed up because they usually develop other com-plications of hypertension.

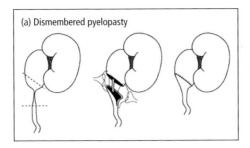

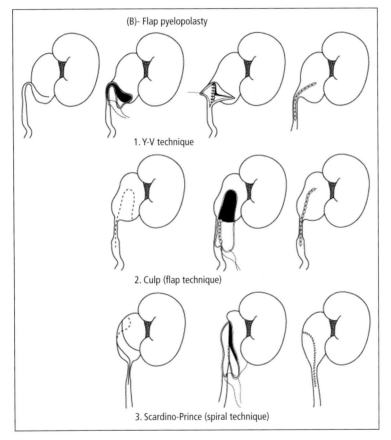

Figure 12.16 Open pyeloplasty.

Ureteric injury

Accidental trauma

Closed injuries of the ureter are very rare. Open injuries caused by a knife or bullet are easily overlooked at the time the wound is explored, and may only be noticed afterwards when urine leaks from the wound.

Iatrogenic trauma

The ureter is at risk in any operation in the pelvis, especially hysterectomy. The ureter is most prone

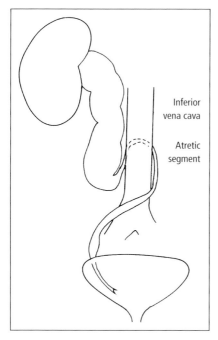

Figure 12.17 Retrocaval ureter.

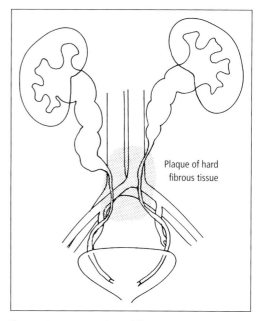

Figure 12.18 Retroperitoneal fibrosis.

to be injured where it is crossed by the uterine arteries and veins, but it can also be caught a little higher up by a suture used to close the peritoneum. There are three distinct clinical scenarios.

Injury noticed at operation

If the ureter is healthy, it may be repaired by end-to-end anastomosis using absorbable sutures and a splint left in.

Immediate postoperative symptoms

1 *Loin pain and fever:* More often the injury to the ureter is not noticed during the operation. The patient may have pain in the loin afterwards, and if the urine is infected, a fever. These are important symptoms demand an immediate IVU.
2 *Anuria:* If both ureters have been obstructed at the time of injury, the patient will be anuric. In practice, the problem arises in just the kind of operation where there is likely to have been considerable loss of blood, and it is reasonable to think

that shock has caused renal failure from underperfusion. When there is any doubt, an IVU should be done: if there is obstruction there will be a delayed nephrogram.

Late leak of urine

Sadly, the pain in the loin is often put down to normal postoperative discomfort. After 7–10 days, fluid begins to escape from the vagina.

First and most urgent task is to confirm that the fluid is urine. This is easy: have it sent to the laboratory for an urgent creatinine measurement. If the creatinine is greater than that in the blood the fluid just has to be urine.

The second step is to get an IVU. This will usually show some obstruction, and occasionally will show extravasation of the contrast into the vagina or soft tissues (Fig. 12.20). Forget the traditional arcane ritual of putting a series of swabs into the vagina or methylene blue into the bladder. These confuse the issue and waste time. Forget the notion that one must delay intervention for 40 days and 40 nights (or some such nonsense). The sooner

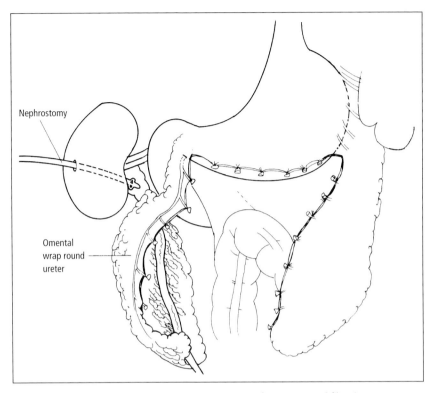

Figure 12.19 Wrapping the ureter in omentum prevents recurrence of retroperitoneal fibrosis.

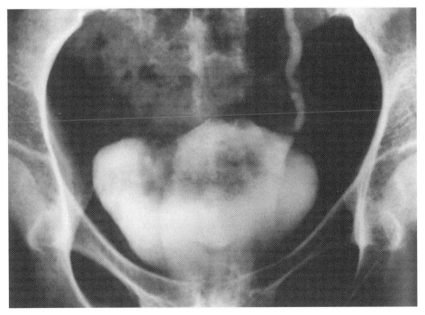

Figure 12.20 IVU in ureterovaginal fistula following hysterectomy: contrast medium outlines the vagina. The ureter is a little obstructed.

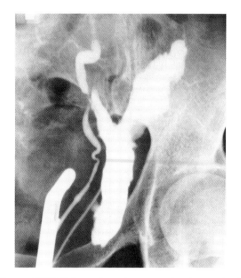

Figure 12.21 Retrograde ureterogram showing contrast leaking out from the ureter.

the diagnosis is confirmed and the injured ureter is repaired the better (and the easier to do).

A bulb-ended catheter is placed in the ureter and contrast injected to give a *ureterogram*. This will show extravasation or a block. It ought to be done on the other side as well since the injury is often bilateral (Fig. 12.21).

Repair of the ureter

The previous incision is reopened. The ureter is traced down to the site of injury, divided where it is healthy, and implanted into a U-shaped (Boari) flap made from the wall of the bladder, with a tunnel to prevent reflux (Fig. 12.22).

Carcinoma of the ureter

Since the ureter is lined with urothelium, it can form all the types of transitional cell cancer that

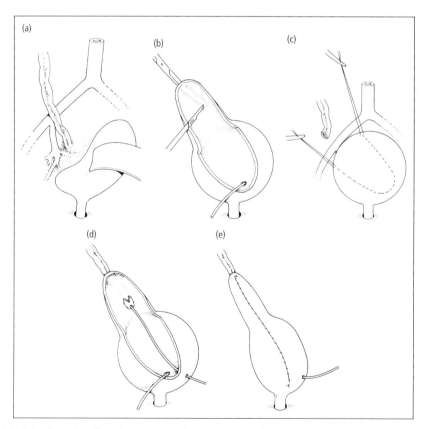

Figure 12.22 Reimplantation of an injured ureter with a Boari bladder flap.

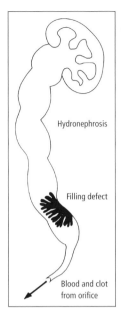

Figure 12.23 Clinical features of a carcinoma of the ureter.

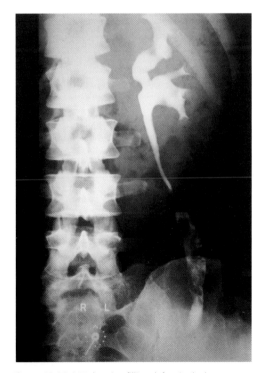

Figure 12.24 IVU showing filling defect in the lower ureter caused by carcinoma.

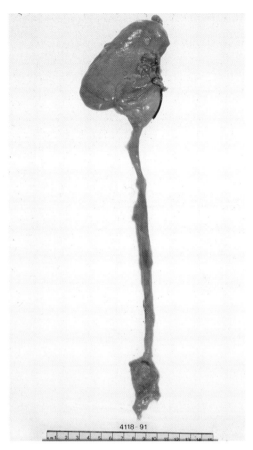

Figure 12.25 Nephroureterectomy specimen showing tumour in the lower ureter and excision of a cuff of the bladder wall.

are seen in the renal pelvis and bladder. They present with haematuria, or pain from obstruction to the ureter (Fig. 12.23).

Diagnosis

The diagnosis is suggested by the IVU, and confirmed by an ureterogram (Fig. 12.24). Malignant cells may be found in the urine on cytology if the tumour is G2 or G3. Ureteroscopy gives a clear picture of the tumour and allows a biopsy to be taken.

Treatment

Single G1 tumours can occasionally be removed locally, or coagulated with a laser through the ureteroscope, but unfortunately they are usually multiple. G3 tumours have a very bad prognosis, and have often invaded through the wall of the ureter by the time they are detected, so that in addition to nephroureterectomy (Fig. 12.25), adjuvant radiotherapy or chemotherapy is usually necessary.

Chapter 13

The bladder: structure and function

Surgical anatomy

In children the bladder is an abdominal organ, easily felt and aspirated. In adults it cannot be felt unless it is distended because it lies deep behind the symphysis. Above, the dome of the bladder is covered by peritoneum, against which lie loops of small bowel and sigmoid colon. A long tail of urachus tethers the dome of the bladder to the umbilicus: this is the vestige of the foetal allantois.

As the bladder becomes distended it rises, not always in the midline, and it may bulge out into the inguinal canal to form the 'bladder ears' often seen in cystograms in normal children. In adults the bladder is just medial to the neck of an inguinal or femoral hernia.

Posteriorly, the bladder is separated from the rectum by the fascia of Denonvilliers which is made of two fused layers of peritoneum. This forms a remarkable biological barrier which prevents carcinoma of the bladder or prostate spreading into the rectum, and acts as a most useful plane of cleavage in radical surgery on the prostate (Fig. 13.1).

In the male the bladder rests on the prostate gland, below which is the levator ani muscle. In

Lecture Notes: Urology, 6th edition. By John Blandy and Amir Kaisary. Published 2009 by Blackwell Publishing. ISBN: 978-1-4051-2270-2.

females the bladder rests on the anterior wall of the vagina (Fig. 13.2).

The fibres of the detrusor muscle of the bladder are not arranged in layers as in the bowel but run criss-cross, like a basket, each fibre passing from outer to inner layers and back again. Unlike most other viscera, the bladder has no capsule; its muscle lies against fat, connective tissue and a plexus of large veins.

The detrusor muscle is lined by a thin layer of submucosa on which lies the waterproof urothelium (Fig. 13.3).

Blood supply

The arteries come from branches of the internal iliac artery of which the largest, the *superior vesical artery*, crosses in front of the ureter (Fig. 13.4). The veins of the bladder drain into the internal iliac veins, but in addition, a second 'backstairs' system drains into the marrow of the pelvic bones, femora and vertebral bodies. Any increase in intra-abdominal pressure forces blood from the bladder into the bone marrow; hence, metastases from cancer of the prostate and bladder are often found there.

The rich network of lymphatics in the deeper layers of the detrusor muscle drains into the lymph nodes of the pelvis. Like the veins, there are also direct communications with the bone marrow of the pelvis, vertebrae and femora.

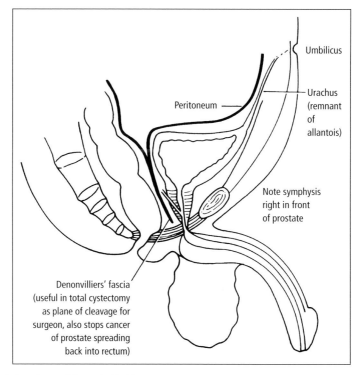

Figure 13.1 Surgical anatomy of the male bladder.

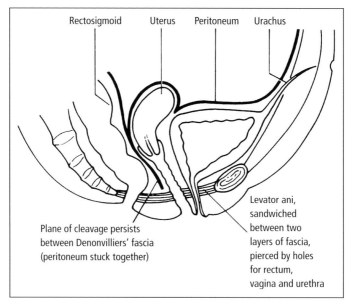

Figure 13.2 Surgical anatomy of the female bladder.

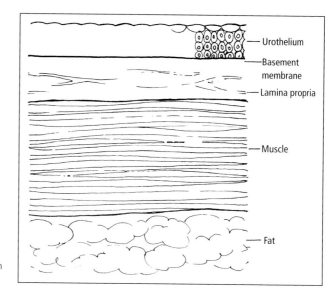

Figure 13.3 Diagram of section through wall of bladder.

Nerves of the bladder

Spinal cord segments

The S2 and S3 segments of the spinal cord lie in the conus medullaris at the level of T12/L1 which is just where the back is most often injured in traffic or industrial accidents.

Afferent

Afferent impulses from the bladder pass up in the pelvic parasympathetic nerves – *nervi erigentes* – to the S2 and S3 segments of the spinal cord. Sensation of *pain* is also conveyed in sympathetic fibres which run via the presacral plexus and lumbar sympathetic ganglia to reach surprisingly

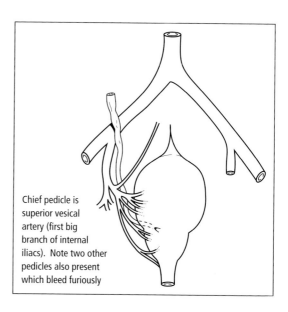

Chief pedicle is superior vesical artery (first big branch of internal iliacs). Note two other pedicles also present which bleed furiously

Figure 13.4 Blood supply of the bladder.

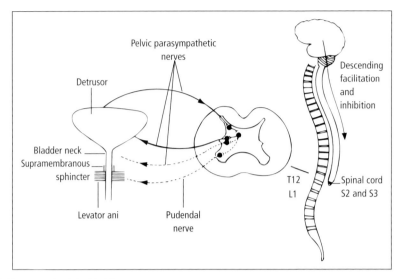

Figure 13.5 Nerve supply of the bladder.

high levels in the spinal cord: indeed to block all pain from the bladder, a spinal anaesthetic must reach as high as T6. The fibres of both sets of autonomic nerves follow the arterial branches to reach the bladder (Fig. 13.5).

Efferent

From the S2 and S3 segments *efferent* motor impulses go to the bladder along three sets of nerves:
1 *parasympathetic* fibres to ganglia in the wall of the detrusor muscle causing it to contract;
2 *sympathetic* fibres to the supramembranous sphincter and the neck of the bladder (alpha-adrenergic receptors); and
3 *somatic myelinated fibres* in the pudendal nerve supply the striated muscle of the levator ani.

Micturition

Filling of the bladder stimulates *stretch receptors* which send impulses up the parasympathetic afferent fibres. The reflex arc in the S2 and S3 segments returns impulses to the detrusor along parasympathetic fibres causing it to contract, and at the same time, inhibits not only the efferent sympathetic impulses going to the bladder neck and

supramembranous sphincter, but also those going in the myelinated fibres of the pudendal nerve to the levator ani and pelvic floor.

When the bladder has been emptied out, first the pelvic floor contracts, then the supramembranous sphincter milks back urine from the upper part of the urethra into the bladder, and finally the bladder neck is closed (Fig. 13.6).

Like all reflexes, that for micturition is modified by influences from higher up in the nervous system which may either facilitate or inhibit the reflex arc. We all are aware that on occasions the urge to empty an overdistended bladder drives all other thoughts from consciousness, and that anxiety or fright may bring on an urge to urinate.

Urodynamics

Cystometry

Through a fine catheter, water is slowly run into the bladder while its pressure (P_{ves}) is continually recorded through a second catheter, introduced either alongside the first in the urethra, or through a small needle inserted suprapubically (Fig. 13.7). A third catheter placed inside the rectum measures intra-abdominal pressure (P_{abd}), and a computer

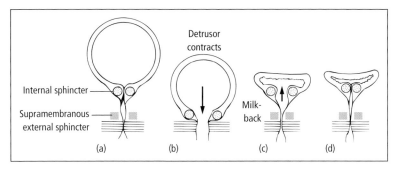

Figure 13.6 Emptying of the bladder.

subtracts this from the intravesical measurement to give the true detrusor pressure (P_{det}) (Fig. 13.8).

The measurements are made while the bladder is filled, and while the patient passes urine into an electronic *flow meter*, a device that automatically records the flow rate (Q_{max}) and the volume of urine that has been collected (V_{comp}) (Fig. 13.9).

Voiding cystometrogram

These measurements can be combined with a video X-ray recording of the *cystogram* by using dilute contrast medium instead of water. Study of the recording allows one to see the bladder neck opening and closing, and to note any reflux of urine up the ureters.

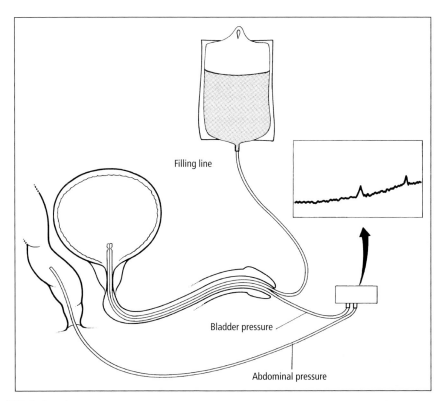

Figure 13.7 Cystometry.

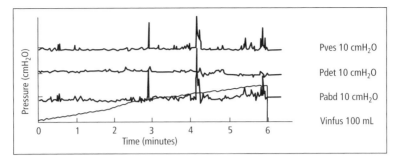

Figure 13.8 Cystometrogram.

Electromyography

The activity of the striated muscle of the levator ani can be recorded from small needle electrodes inserted into the muscle. This is not a routine investigation and calls for considerable experience in its use and interpretation. At rest there is normally a constant level of activity in the levator ani, which, when the electromyogram is connected to a loudspeaker, sounds like a constant buzz. While the bladder is emptying and the impulses down the pudendal nerve are inhibited, there should be silence (Fig. 13.10).

Urethral pressure profile

The pressure inside the lumen of the urethra can be measured with a catheter that is withdrawn at a constant rate along the urethra. The pressure is drawn on a graph which measures the distance along the urethra, giving the urethral pressure profile. This is not a routine investigation, but is of help in some cases of incontinence (Fig. 13.11).

Cystoscopy

Flexible cystoscopy

Fine glass fibres are flexible. If made of completely clear optical glass, and coated with glass of a different refractive index; the entire light entering one end will leave the other (Fig. 13.12). A large number of these fibres are wound on a wheel, glued at one spot, and cut through. The result is a fibre-optic cable which can be introduced into any orifice of the body, and will transmit an image in a series of tiny dots like ground glass (Fig. 13.13).

The modern flexible cystoscope has channels for irrigation, for light, and for passing flexible instruments such as biopsy forceps, laser fibres or

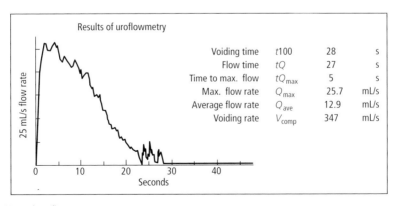

Figure 13.9 Normal uroflow measurement.

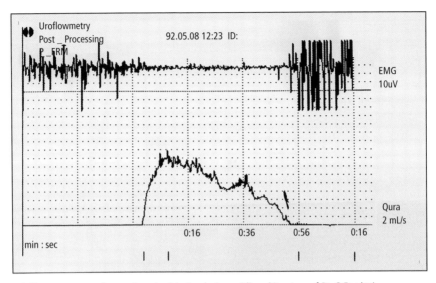

Figure 13.10 Electromyogram from external sphincter during voiding. (Courtesy of Dr C Fowler.)

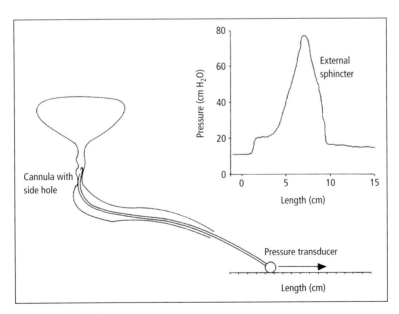

Figure 13.11 Urethral pressure profile.

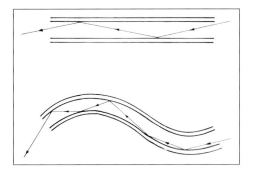

Figure 13.12 Total internal reflection along a glass fibre.

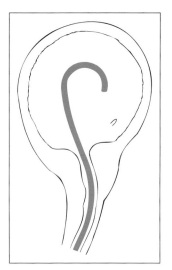

Figure 13.14 The flexible cystoscope can give a view of the trigone and bladder neck.

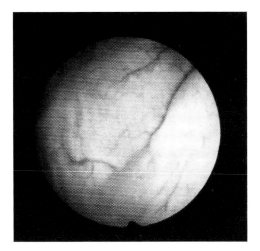

Figure 13.13 Image obtained through flexible cystoscope.

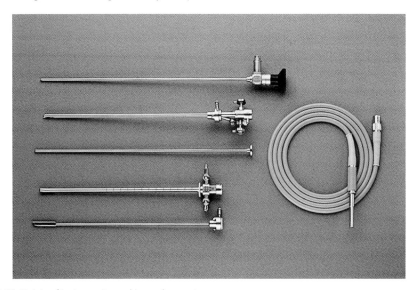

Figure 13.15 Variety of instruments used in modern cystoscopy.

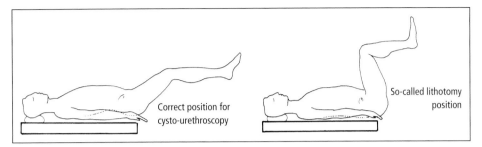

Correct position for
cysto-urethroscopy

So-called lithotomy
position

Figure 13.16 Correct position for cystoscopy.

a diathermy electrode. Passing the cystoscope is painless. It is gently advanced along the urethra under vision as water is slowly run in. After examining the urethra, sphincter, prostatic urethra and bladder neck, the inside of the bladder is carefully inspected. By bending the cystoscope back on itself the bladder neck and prostate can be viewed from inside (Fig. 13.14). Flexible cystoscopy is usually done in the outpatient clinic/day surgery units which is very convenient for the majority of patients and is cost effective.

Rigid cystoscope

The image seen through the rigid cystoscope is much clearer than that of the flexible instrument, and the instrument channel allows a large variety of gadgets to be used inside the bladder (Fig. 13.15). Biopsies can be taken, tumours resected, stones crushed, ureters catheterised and examined. It is less comfortable for the patient than the flexible cystoscopy, and for some of these manoeuvres a general or spinal anaesthetic is required. The patient is placed in the cystoscopy position (Fig. 13.16).

Technological advances are being made all the time to improve the instruments and give better vision. Attaching a camera to the telescope eyepiece saves the urologist 'bending' down to look into the telescope saving untoward physical strain on his neck. Using the camera allows projection of the view on large screens which is valuable in teaching members of staff. It also allows photography and video recording for record keeping and exchange of information.

Chapter 14

The bladder: congenital abnormalities and trauma

Congenital abnormalities

During the complicated process of the bladder embryological evolution, the foetal hindgut, the cloaca, curls round. Its tip becomes the urachus, and the urogenital septum comes down to separate the future bladder from the rectum. It brings with it the mesonephric ducts which sprout the ureters (Fig. 14.1). There are many opportunities for things to go wrong, and a variety of congenital abnormalities may occur:

1 *Agenesis:* The cloaca may not form at all; both ureters are obstructed, and the condition is not compatible with survival.

2 *Duplication:* Very rarely the bladder is divided by a septum either in the midline or lying transversely.

3 *Patent urachus:* If there is obstruction at the neck of the bladder or the urethra the urachus may remain patent and leak urine at the umbilicus. Cysts may form in the remnant of the urachus and may become infected in later life. Because the urachus is a remnant of the hindgut, and is lined with bowel epithelium, it can give rise to an adenocarcinoma. This presents with haematuria, and on cystoscopy a small red lump like a cherry is seen at the apex of the bladder which is always much smaller than the mass which can be felt outside (Fig. 14.2).

4 *Exstrophy:* In early foetal life the cloacal membrane may extend up to the umbilicus, and prevent the ingrowth of the future abdominal wall. Normally the cloacal membrane dissolves only at the site of the future anus, vagina and urethra. In exstrophy it exposes tissue below the umbilicus varying in extent from a dorsal cleft in the penis – epispadias – to the entire cloaca. In the most common variety, the bladder opens like a flat red patch on the abdomen onto which the ureters discharge urine. This is often accompanied by a prolapse of the rectum, undescended testes, and wide separation of the symphysis pubis (Fig. 14.3).

Untreated, the condition is miserable. The child is continually soaked in urine. The exposed urothelium is always irritated, painful and inflamed, and eventually may undergo glandular metaplasia which in time goes on to develop adenocarcinoma. All this can be prevented.

Firstly, it is important to reassure the distraught parents that all will be well. Secondly, transfer the baby to a specialist paediatric unit where the operation to close the bladder is performed as soon as possible after birth. The bladder is mobilised, sewn into a sphere, and the abdominal wall closed over it. The sacroiliac joints may be divided to allow the pelvis to be closed like an

Lecture Notes: Urology, 6th edition. By John Blandy and Amir Kaisary. Published 2009 by Blackwell Publishing. ISBN: 978-1-4051-2270-2.

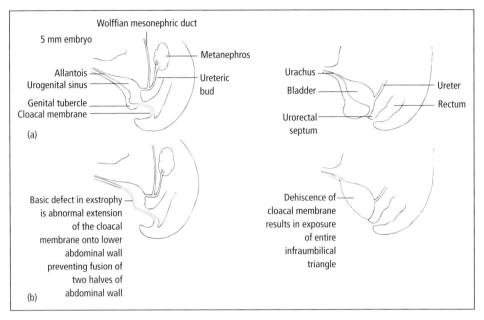

Figure 14.1 Embryological evolution of the bladder and the role of the cloacal membrane in the cause of exstrophy.

oyster (Fig. 14.4). Additional operations will be required later to reconstruct the bladder neck to restore continence, to reconstruct the penis, and to bring down the testicles. Eventually these children grow up to lead a normal life: the boys have a normal sex life, and the girls can have children.

5 *Epispadias:* In this minor version of exstrophy, the urethra opens on the proximal end of the dorsum of a short, flat penis which curves upwards (Fig. 14.5). This can also be completely refashioned in expert hands: first a new urethra is formed, and later the bladder neck is reconstructed to restore continence.

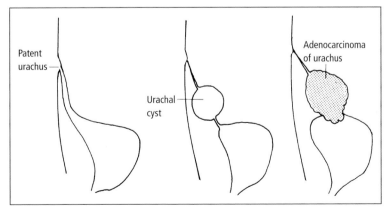

Figure 14.2 Disorders of the persistent urachus.

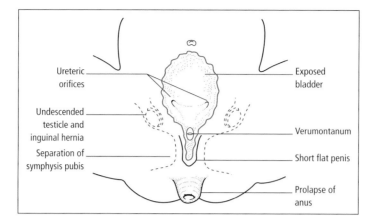

Figure 14.3 Exstrophy.

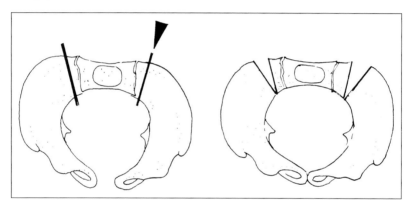

Figure 14.4 Iliac osteotomy to assist closure of exstrophy.

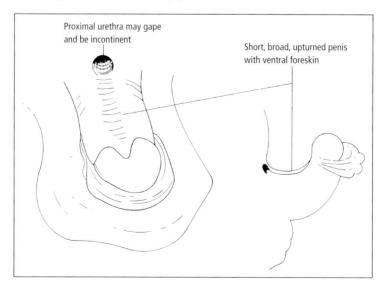

Figure 14.5 Epispadias.

Trauma

Open and penetrating injuries

The bladder may be injured in any penetrating abdominal injury. It is closed with absorbable sutures and a catheter is left in for about a week. The same management is used when the bladder is opened in the course of some abdominal operation. The outcome is a perfectly functioning bladder.

One new type of penetrating injury has recently become of importance: people with a patch of small intestine added on to the bladder to increase its capacity or cure detrusor instability often have to catheterise themselves, and from time to time the catheter may perforate the bladder. The clinical features are those of a delayed perforation (see below).

Closed injury: intraperitoneal rupture

The typical patient is run over while he lies drunk with a distended bladder (Fig. 14.6). The bladder bursts and a large volume of urine enters the peritoneal cavity but it is dilute and does not at first

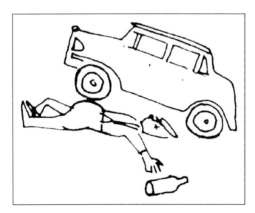

Figure 14.6 Closed injury to the bladder.

cause any chemical irritation. Only after several hours does the patient become ill.

Diagnosis

1 *Paracentesis:* If there is some reason to think there may be other intra-abdominal injuries, a four-quadrant tap is performed. If this shows blood, laparotomy or laparoscopy is performed and if a tear is found in the bladder, it is repaired with absorbable sutures and a catheter left in the bladder.
2 *Cystogram:* A cystogram may show contrast leaking into the peritoneal cavity, but only if the bladder is fully distended.
3 *Cystoscopy:* A flexible cystoscopy will show the tear.

Treatment

If there is no evidence of peritonitis an indwelling catheter is left in the bladder for about a week, and then tested with a cystogram to show that the tear has healed.

Delayed perforation

After coagulation of a small recurrent cancer in the bladder, the necrotic wall of the bladder may give way about a week later, and allow urine to leak into the peritoneal cavity. Typically there is very little pain, and there are almost no abnormal physical signs at first, but after a few hours the abdomen becomes distended and the bowel sounds can no longer be heard. Paracentesis will yield evil smelling fluid. If detected early, the condition is relieved by keeping the bladder emptied with a catheter, but if there is any doubt, or if the patient's condition is not improving, laparotomy, evacuation of the fluid and repair of the lacerated bladder is the safest course.

Chapter 15

Urinary tract infection

Urinary tract infection (UTI) is a broad term used to describe microbial colonisation of the urine. It includes infection of the structures of the urinary tract from the kidney down to the urethral meatus. Infection of organs such as the prostate and epididymis are also included in the definition.

Bacteriuria denotes the presence of bacteria in the urine, which is usually free of bacteria. It can be symptomatic or asymptomatic. Pyuria is the presence of white blood cells (WBCs) in the urine and is generally accepted as an indication of infection and as an inflammatory response of the urothelium to the bacteria. It is to be noted that bacteriuria without pyuria is an indication of bacterial colonisation of the urinary tract without infection. Such sterile pyuria would warrant consideration of other pathological conditions, including tuberculosis, stone disease or cancer.

Uncomplicated UTI is a term describing infection in healthy patients who have a structurally and functionally normal urinary tract. Complicated UTI is usually associated with elements which increase the chances of acquiring bacteria and decreasing treatment efficacy. Risk factors for complicated UTI include anatom-

ical and functional urinary tract abnormalities, pregnancy, old age, diabetes, immunosuppression, urinary tract instrumentation and indwelling catheters.

UTI can affect both females and males, including the newly born, infants and young children. UTI in women is common and the incidence increases with age. Sexually active women are at the highest risk.

Pathogenesis

Most UTIs are caused by anaerobic bacteria, usually from the bowel flora. Gram-negative bacteria include *Escherichia coli* (by far the most common), *Proteus*, and *Klebsiella*. Gram-positive bacteria include *E. faecalis* and *S. saprophyticus*.

Bacterial virulence factors play a role in determining which bacteria invade the urinary system, and determine the extent of infection. Bacterial adherence to vaginal and urothelial epithelial cells is an essential step in the initiation of UTI. It has been noted that some women have recurrent UTI/cystitis at regular intervals possibly linked to oestrogen levels. In postmenopausal women, where there are lowered oestrogen levels, the incidence of UTI can be decreased by oestrogen replacement therapy. Alterations to host defensive mechanisms are to be noted when causes of UTI are addressed. These include obstruction, prostate enlargement in men, urethral stenosis in women,

Lecture Notes: Urology, 6th edition. By John Blandy and Amir Kaisary. Published 2009 by Blackwell Publishing. ISBN: 978-1-4051-2270-2.

vesicoureteric reflux, diabetes mellitus, human immunodeficiency virus and spinal cord injuries with high-pressure bladders.

Urine specimen collection

The correct collection of a urine specimen is important. In men, the glans penis is carefully cleaned and, during reasonably forceful urination, initial, mid-stream and terminal specimens can be collected in separate containers. In women, cleanliness in collection of urine specimens is important and attention must be focused on avoiding contamination. In the sitting position, and with the labia held apart with two fingers from one hand, it is possible to collect a specimen of urine without touching the skin. In infants and young children, the penis or female pudendum is cleaned in a similar manner as with adults. Urination can be stimulated by pressure over the suprapubic area or stroking of the paraspinal muscles to elicit the Perez reflex. In some cases catheterisation or a suprapubic tap are necessary.

If urine is to be cultured, but cannot be cultured within 4 hours of collection, the sample should be refrigerated or preserved with boric acid immediately. Inspection of infected urine shows it to be cloudy; crystal clear urine is never infected. It smells fishy. Microscopy shows it to be full of pus cells (more than 5 per high power field) and bacteria can be seen along the edge of the leucocytes (Fig. 15.1). The urine is cultured at once using a dip-slide, or cooled and sent as soon as possible to a laboratory where a colony count is performed and antibiotic sensitivities are determined.

Different types of UTI and associated disorders

UTIs are often discussed clinically by their presumed site of origin, behaviour pattern or both. In addition to the prescription of antibiotics, where indicated, making the urine alkaline by giving up to 6 g sodium bicarbonate per day, or a similar amount of potassium citrate, and keeping the

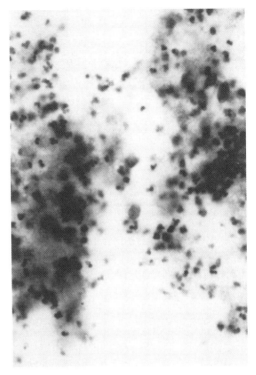

Figure 15.1 Pus in the urine. (Courtesy of Professor Jo Martin.)

urine dilute by drinking 3 L of fluid a day makes urination less painful.

Simple cystitis

Acute cystitis involves only the lower urinary tract; it is an inflammation of the bladder due to bacterial or nonbacterial causes (i.e. radiation, viral). Patients with cystitis may present with a variety of symptoms, including urinary frequency, urgency, dysuria and suprapubic pain (Fig 15.2). It occurs in approximately 1% of pregnant women, of whom 60% have a negative result on initial screening. In females, acute cystitis is common and usually innocent. Bloody urine is reported in as many as 10% of cases of UTI in otherwise healthy women; this condition is called haemorrhagic cystitis. In males, acute cystitis usually signifies an important underlying disorder and needs thorough investigation. Bacterial cystitis without concomitant

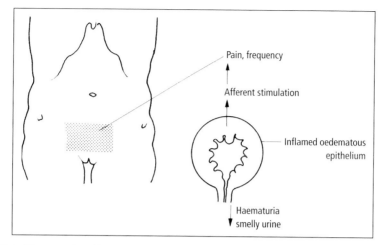

Figure 15.2 Clinical features of cystitis.

infection in other portions of the genitourinary tract is believed to be rare in males. The abrupt onset of irritative voiding symptoms (e.g. frequency, urgency, nocturia, dysuria) and suprapubic pain are clinically diagnostic. Symptoms alone do not distinguish cystitis (lower UTI) from pyelonephritis (upper UTI). Although simple lower UTI (cystitis) may resolve spontaneously, effective treatment lessens the duration of symptoms and reduces the incidence of progression to upper UTI.

Uncomplicated cystitis should be treated for 3 days. A 7-day course of appropriate antimicrobial therapy is recommended in patients who have had symptoms for 1 week or more, those with complicating factors, and in men.

Like a dustbin, the bladder only stays clean if it is emptied regularly (Fig. 15.3). Even when the last drop of urine has been expelled, some bacteria cling to the urothelial cells after the bladder has been emptied. Normally these are easily dealt with by the natural bactericidal action of the urothelial cells, but this function is impaired in diabetes and in cancer cells. Deliberate infection of the bladder with an inoculum of microbes does not cause an infection if the bladder is emptied regularly. However, if the bladder does not empty out completely, because of outflow obstruction or a diverticulum, then a tiny inoculum will divide at body temperature to become millions.

Pathology of chronic cystitis

Follicular cystitis: Here repeated infections give rise to collections of lymphocytes under the urothelium which can be recognised as pale specks on cystoscopy (Fig. 15.4).

Cystitis cystica: In severe infections parts of the urothelium are shed, leaving islands of cells which get buried under the regenerating urothelium: these form little cysts under the mucosa which look like little bubbles on cystoscopy – cystitis cystica. This is usually harmless, but if the infection persists, the buried cysts of urothelium undergo metaplasia,

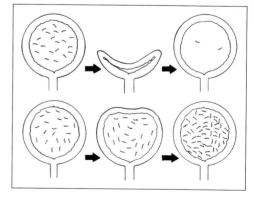

Figure 15.3 The chief defence of the bladder against infection is to keep itself regularly emptied out completely.

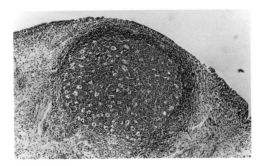

Figure 15.4 Cystitis follicularis.

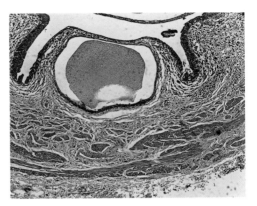

Figure 15.5 Cystitis cystica.

secrete mucus, and turn into intestinal mucosa – adenomatous metaplasia – which may be the precursor of adenocarcinoma (Fig. 15.5).

Malacoplakia: A variation on this theme is malacoplakia, which forms collections of soft brown lumps in the urothelium which are easily mistaken for cancer.

Squamous metaplasia: Persistent infection, especially when associated with a stone, stricture or schistosomiasis, causes the urothelium to undergo squamous metaplasia. This is very sinister because it often progresses to squamous cell cancer.

Alkaline encrusted cystitis: Infection with *Proteus mirabilis* can lead to a peculiarly disabling condition in which chronic inflammation accompanied by calcification involves the entire wall of the bladder, converting it into a rigid sphere. Cystoscopy shows stony encrustation all over the wall of the bladder. The urine reeks of ammonia.

Pyelonephritis

Patients with pyelonephritis are generally diagnosed based upon their clinical presentation. The classic presentation of fever chills and costovertebral angle tenderness is frequently seen on physical examination. Patients may also experience nausea, vomiting, diarrhoea and/or irritative voiding symptoms. Along with positive urine cultures, excessive numbers of white blood cells, sometimes in casts, as well as red blood cells are found in the urine. Blood cultures may also be positive, and serum studies may reveal an elevated erythrocyte sedimentation rate and elevations in C-reactive protein and/or creatinine. Acute pyelonephritis can lead to septicaemia and is best treated initially by injection of a broad-spectrum antibacterial such as cefuroxime or a quinolone especially if the patient is severely ill; gentamicin can also be used. Therapy should be tailored to the patient. In a patient without complicating factors, outpatient therapy with an oral fluoroquinolone or trimethoprim–sulfamethoxazole (TMP-SMX) is effective. In patients who appear ill or are unable to tolerate oral therapy due to nausea or vomiting and warrant hospitalisation, therapy with a parenteral fluoroquinolone, aminoglycoside (with or without ampicillin), or an extended spectrum cephalosporin is advisable. The recommended duration of treatment is 7–14 days. Many patients have intermittent fevers and flank pain despite appropriate anti-microbial therapy, but these symptoms typically resolve after 72 hours. Imaging is indicated when the patient does not respond after 3 days. Repeat urine cultures should be obtained after 5–7 days of therapy, and again 4–6 weeks later, to ensure sterility. Up to 30% of patients may relapse after 14 days of treatment but are usually cured by a repeat 14-day course of appropriate antimicrobial therapy.

Recurrent UTI reinfections

Recurrent UTIs with new infections from bacteria outside the urinary tract should be distinguished from cases of persistent bacteria within the urinary tract. Recurrent infections often occur in women and girls secondary to ascending colonisation from faecal flora. In healthy women, further work-up is not required. However, imaging studies and cystoscopy should be considered in women with evidence of upper tract infections, obstructive symptoms, unexplained haematuria, suspected neurogenic bladder, multiple sclerosis or diabetes mellitus.

Postmenopausal women also appear to have an increased risk of recurrent UTI due to changes in vaginal flora, and vaginal oestrogen cream should be considered as a preventative measure. Women are also at risk.

Long-term low-dose therapy may be required in selected patients to prevent recurrence of infection; indications include frequent relapses and significant kidney damage. Trimethoprim, nitrofurantoin and cefalexin have been recommended for long-term therapy.

Depending on the clinical scenario, prophylaxis can be continuous or post-intercourse. The mechanism of action of trimethoprim or TMP-SMX is via elimination of gut colonisation. Nitrofurantoin, however, does not alter gut flora, and faecal and vaginal flora remain unchanged. It is associated with adverse reactions, including pulmonary and allergic reactions, the risk of which increases in patients over 50 years of age.

Complicated UTI

These cases include those that occur in patients with a compromised urinary tract system, or those caused by very resistant bacteria. The clinical variations range from mild cystitis to life-threatening urinary sepsis. Urine analysis, culture and sensitivity are mandatory. Radiological and non-invasive scanning tools are usually necessary to evaluate any underlying urinary tract abnormalities and should be employed. As there are no adequate guidelines for antibiotic therapy in such cases, broad-spectrum antibiotics with excellent urinary and tissue levels and safety profile should be utilised.

Unresolved UTI bacterial resistance

Microbes are now emerging that are resistant to cheap and effective first-line drugs. Bacteria are particularly efficient at developing resistance, not only because of their ability to multiply very rapidly but also because they can transfer their resistance genes when the bacteria replicate. Infections caused by resistant microbes fail to respond to treatment, resulting in prolonged illness. This resistance has come about from both over- and under-use of antibiotics: physicians have prescribed antimicrobials in the absence of appropriate indications or over-prescribed broad-spectrum injectable agents when a narrow-spectrum oral agent would have been more appropriate. Conversely, patients forget to take medication or interrupt their treatment when they begin to feel better, thereby creating an ideal environment for microbes to adapt rather than be killed. Widespread bacterial resistance, especially to ampicillin, amoxicillin and trimethoprim, has increased the importance of urine culture before therapy.

To prevent the creation of resistant microbes, it is best to start with a safe and cheap antimicrobial, e.g. trimethoprim, nitrofurantoin or nalidixic acid. Reserve expensive wide-spectrum antibiotics for severe cases, and use them under microbiological control. A patient who has suffered previous attacks will know which antimicrobial agent made them better last time, and it is sensible to use it again, pending sensitivity studies from the laboratory. While awaiting culture results, empiric treatment with fluoroquinolone may be appropriate in patients whose symptoms are severe.

The UK Health Protection Agency advises prescribing an antibiotic only when there is likely to be a clear clinical benefit. Other recommendations include avoiding broad spectrum antibiotics (e.g. co-amoxiclav, quinolones and cephalosporins) when standard and less expensive antibiotics remain effective, as they increase the risk of *Clostridium difficile*, MRSA and resistant UTIs. Amoxicillin resistance is common; therefore, only use this if a culture confirms susceptibility. Do not treat asymptomatic bacteriuria in the elderly; it is not

Table 15.1 NICE guideline for UTI in children.

Age group	Symptoms and signs		
	Most common to least common		
Infants younger than 3 months	Fever	Poor feeding	Abdominal pain
	Vomiting	Failure to thrive	Jaundice
	Lethargy		Haematuria
	Irritability		Offensive urine
Infants and children, 3 months or older			
Preverbal	Fever	Abdominal pain	Lethargy
		Loin tenderness	Irritability
		Vomiting	Haematuria
		Poor feeding	Offensive urine
			Failure to thrive
Verbal	Frequency	Dysfunctional voiding	Fever
	Dysuria	Changes to continence	Malaise
		Abdominal pain	Vomiting
		Loin tenderness	Haematuria
			Offensive urine
			Cloudy urine

associated with increased morbidity. In the presence of a catheter, antibiotics will not eradicate bacteriuria; only treat if the patient is systemically unwell or if pyelonephritis seems likely.

Alternative treatments for resistant organisms suggested by the British National Formulary include co-amoxiclav (amoxicillin with clavulanic acid), an oral cephalosporin, pivmecillinam or a quinolone.

NICE guideline for UTI in children

UTI is a common bacterial infection in infants and children. It may be difficult to recognise because the presenting symptoms and signs are non-specific, particularly in infants and children younger than 3 years.

Symptoms and signs

Table 15.1 is a guide to the symptoms and signs infants and children may present:

1 Infants and children presenting with an unexplained fever of 38°C or other symptoms suggestive of a UTI should have a urine sample tested.

The following risk factors for UTI and serious underlying pathology should be recorded:

- poor urine flow;
- history suggesting previous UTI or confirmed previous UTI;
- recurrent fever of uncertain origin;
- antenatally diagnosed renal abnormality;
- family history of vesicoureteric reflux or renal disease;
- constipation;
- dysfunctional voiding;
- enlarged bladder;
- abdominal mass;
- evidence of spinal lesion;
- poor growth; and
- high blood pressure.

2 Infants and children who have bacteriuria and fever of 38°C should be considered to have acute pyelonephritis/upper UTI.

3 Infants and children presenting with fever of <38°C with loin pain/tenderness and bacteriuria should also be considered to have acute pyelonephritis/upper UTI. All other infants and children who have bacteriuria but no systemic symptoms or signs should be considered to have cystitis/lower UTI.

Acute management

Early recognition and prompt treatment of UTIs are important to prevent progression of infection to pyelonephritis or urosepsis and to avoid late sequelae such as renal scarring or renal failure.

1 Infants younger than 3 months with a possible UTI should be referred immediately to the care of a paediatric specialist.

2 For infants and children 3 months or older with acute pyelonephritis/upper UTI:

- Consider referral to a paediatric specialist.
- Treat with oral antibiotics for 7–10 days. The use of an oral antibiotic with low resistance patterns is recommended, for example cephalosporin or co-amoxiclav.
- If oral antibiotics cannot be used, treat with an intravenous antibiotic agent such as cefotaxime or ceftriaxone for 2–4 days followed by oral antibiotics for a total duration of 10 days.

3 For infants and children 3 months or older with cystitis/lower UTI:

- Treat with oral antibiotics for 3 days. The choice of antibiotics should be directed by locally developed multidisciplinary guidance. Trimethoprim, nitrofurantoin, cephalosporin or amoxicillin may be suitable.
- Parents or carers should be advised to bring the infant or child for reassessment if the infant or child is still unwell after 24–48 hours. If an alternative diagnosis is not made, a urine sample should be sent for culture to identify the presence of bacteria and determine antibiotic sensitivity if urine culture has not already been carried out.

Start antibiotics after urinalysis and culture are obtained. Do not use short-course therapy in children because it is more difficult to differentiate cystitis from pyelonephritis. An exception is the use of short-course therapy in adolescent females with classic cystitis.

Scottish Intercollegiate Guidelines Network

Management of suspected bacterial UTI in adults has been recommended in a national clinical guideline (Table 15.2).

Table 15.2 Scottish Intercollegiate Guidelines Network (SIGN): Management of suspected bacterial urinary tract infection in adults – a national clinical guideline.

Symptoms of UTI include:
Dysuria
Urgency
Frequency
Polyuria
Suprapubic tenderness
Fever
Flank or back pain

Signs of upper UTI include:
Loin pain
Flank tenderness
Fever
Rigors
Other manifestations of systematic inflammatory response

Diagnosis and treatment of UTI

In women

In otherwise healthy women presenting with symptoms or signs of a UTI, treatment with an antibiotic should be considered. If dysuria and urinary frequency are both present, the probability of UTI is >90%. In women with symptoms of vaginal itch or discharge, explore alternative diagnoses and consider pelvic examination. Women with limited signs of UTI (no more than two symptoms) should have a dipstick test performed to diagnose bacteriuria. If the test is negative for leucocyte esterase and nitrate, empirical antibiotic treatment should be offered. If a woman remains symptomatic after a single course of treatment, she should be investigated for other potential causes. In elderly patients (>65 years), diagnosis should be based on a full clinical assessment, including vital signs.

Symptomatic bacteriuria occurs in 17–20% of pregnancies, and a standard quantitative urine culture should be routinely performed at the first antenatal visit. Bacteriuria should be confirmed with a second urine culture.

Non-pregnant women with symptoms or signs of acute lower UTI and either a high probability of, or proven bacteriuria, should be treated with trimethoprim or nitrofurantoin for 3 days. If the response to this treatment is not adequate, a urine culture should be taken to guide the next choice of antibiotic.

Non-pregnant women with symptoms or signs of acute upper UTI should be treated with ciprofloxin for 7 days. A urine culture should be taken before treatment is started, to guide treatment choice if the response to this treatment is not adequate. Alternative treatments include cotrimoxazole, pivmecillinam, coamoxiclav and cefixime.

Non-pregnant women with asymptomatic bacteriuria, including those >65 years, should not receive antibiotic treatment.

Women with recurrent UTI should be advised to take cranberry products to reduce the frequency of recurrence.

Pregnant women with symptomatic UTI or asymptomatic bacteriuria should be given an antibiotic. Some antibiotics should not be used during pregnancy due to their effects on the foetus. These include tetracyclines (adverse effects on foetal teeth and bones, congenital defects), quinolones (various congenital defects), trimethoprim in the first trimester (facial defects, cardiac abnormalities), and chloramphenicol and sulfonamides in the last trimester (Gray syndrome; haemolytic anaemia in mothers with glucose-6-phosphate dehydrogenase [G-6-PD] deficiency, jaundice and kernicterus, respectively). Trimethoprim is a folate antagonist. In some women low folate levels have been associated with an increased risk of malformations. However, in women with normal folate status, who are well nourished, therapeutic use of trimethoprim for a short period is unlikely to induce folate deficiency. A number of retrospective reviews and case reports indicate that there is no increased risk of foetal toxicity following exposure to nitrofurantoin during pregnancy. Check the British National Formulary to ensure the antibiotic is not toxic in pregnancy.

In men

All men with symptoms of a UTI should have a urine sample cultured. In men older than 50 years,

the incidence of UTI rises dramatically because of enlargement of the prostate, prostatism and subsequent instrumentation of the urinary tract. In men with a history of fever or back pain, upper UTI should be considered. Differential diagnoses include prostatitis, chlaymidial infection and epididymitis.

Bacterial UTI should be treated with a 2-week course of quinolone. Alternative treatments include trimethoprim, deoxycycline and coamoxiclav. Patients who do not respond to treatment should be investigated for prostatitis. Elderly men (>65 years) with asymptomatic bacteriuria should not receive antibiotic treatment. Patients with symptoms of upper UTI, recurrent UTI or those who fail to respond to appropriate antibiotics should be referred for urological investigation.

> **Key message**
>
> UTI is a common problem which can be at times challenging. It can be easily managed provided there is clear understanding of a simple clinical framework. Careful assessment of the clinical categories and identifying the possible underlying causative factors is essential. The choice of antibiotics available, used sensibly, can be the basis of a successful clinical outcome. Guidelines for the treatment of children and of adults have been released by NICE and SIGN, respectively. Simple antibiotics such as trimethoprim and nitrofurantoin are first-line treatment for most symptomatic UTIs, and their use will also help reduce the occurrence of bacterial resistance.

Interstitial cystitis – Hunner's ulcer

The cause of this strange condition is still unknown. Clinically, the patient, usually a middle-aged woman, has intense pain whenever the bladder is half-filled. The pain is often felt in one place. There is severe frequency. Cystoscopy at first shows no abnormality, but after the bladder has been filled, and the water is allowed to run out, the urothelium seems to be cracked, and blood trickles out – cascade haemorrhage.

Biopsy shows chronic inflammation of the urothelium and the underlying submucosa. It has been suggested (but not proved) that excess of mast cells are present which secrete histamine.

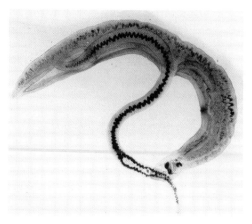

Figure 15.6 *Schistosoma haematobium:* pair of adult worms removed from a vein Schistosomes (about 1 cm long).

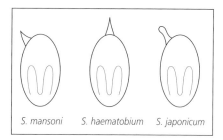

Figure 15.7 Bilharzia ova.

Every year there is a new remedy for this condition but a consistently reliable treatment remains elusive. Some patients are improved if the bladder is stretched; others are better if the 'ulcer' is diathermised; others improve if dimethylsulphoxide is instilled. The condition usually comes back, and the only remedy may be to remove the entire bladder, replacing it with some form of cystoplasty.

Investigations

Every patient with chronic cystitis must be investigated by repeated urine cultures, including those for *Mycobacterium tuberculosis*, by intravenous urogram and cystoscopy to rule out some mechanical cause for persistent infection. In patients who have travelled in Africa the urine should be examined for the ova of *Schistosoma*. Any cause of stagnation in the urinary tract such as a diverticulum, and any local cause for persistent infection such as a stone or necrosis in a tumour must be carefully ruled out.

Treatment

Having excluded remediable causes such as a pocket of undrained urine, a stone, tuberculosis or cancer, then we are left with a large number of patients, usually women, with persistent urinary infection. What can be done for them?

A high fluid throughput often helps dramatically, e.g. 3–4 L/day. This must be combined with frequent emptying of the bladder at least every 2 hours. Busy women should keep a jug of water on their desk and urinate every 2 hours by the clock whether they want to go or not.

This simple, if boring, advice will reduce the number of attacks. But when resistance is low, there will be reinfection. Patients who have had many attacks always know when another is coming on, and they also know which medication is likely to cure them. There is no need to withhold treatment until the laboratory has confirmed what the patient already knows: it is far more sensible to supply your patient with a simple antimicrobial, e.g. trimethoprim or nitrofurantoin, to take whenever an attack threatens. This will often nip the episode in the bud, and she will be cured within 24 hours; if so, there is no need to continue medication any longer.

When this simple system does not work a patient may be given long-term methenamine mandelate or hippurate to reinforce their natural defences.

Schistomiasis (Bilharziasis)

The trematode flukes *Schistosoma haematobium*, *S. mansoni* and *S. japonicum* are flatworms with a life cycle that involves one stage in a mollusc and another in a vertebrate. The adult flukes are about 5 mm in length and live inside human veins, attached to the endothelium by a sucker (Fig. 15.6). The male enfolds the female in a long slit down his belly – hence the name *schisto* (split) and *soma* (body). They were discovered in the portal vein of

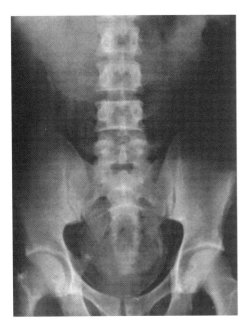

Figure 15.8 Plain X-ray in schistosomiasis showing calcification in the bladder.

children by the German pathologist Theodor Bilharz when he was working in Cairo – hence the alternative name bilharziasis. The females lay eggs with terminal spines which vary according to the species (Fig. 15.7).

When the adult flukes are living in the submucosal veins of the bladder their eggs not only bore their way through the urothelium to cause haematuria, but they cause ulceration and polyp formation. The dead eggs calcify, and can be seen on cystoscopy to glisten like grains of sand under the urothelium. The urothelium undergoes squamous metaplasia and eventually may form squamous cell cancer.

A plain X-ray shows the outline of the bladder, lower ureters and vasa deferentia, traced by the millions of dead calcified ova (Fig. 15.8). Low power microscopy of the urine shows the ova.

If the patient urinates into a slow-moving river or irrigation channel, the eggs hatch into *miracidia* which are attracted to fresh-water snails, which

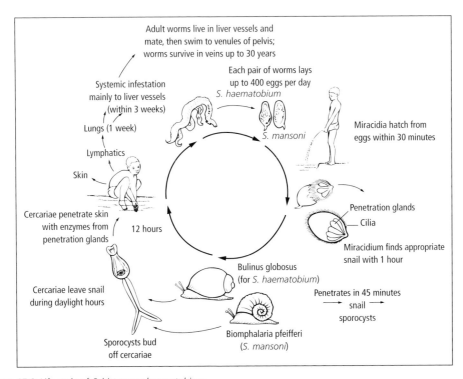

Figure 15.9 Life cycle of *Schistosoma haematobium*.

they invade. They divide inside the body of the snail, form sporocysts which burst to liberate thousands of minute flukes – *cercariae*. These penetrate the skin of any unwary human whose hand or foot happens to be in the water at the right time. It only takes a few seconds for them to enter the skin (Fig. 15.9).

Under the skin, the cercariae cause an itching rash – swimmer's itch. Later they reach the circulation through the lymphatics, and cause a systemic illness – *Katagama fever*. Finally, adult flukes settle in little veins, which may be anywhere in the body including the brain and spinal cord. In small children large masses congregate and obstruct the portal vein. Schistosomiasis is second only to malaria as a cause of disease and its eradication depends on the provision of clean water and effective disposal of sewage.

Treatment

It is futile to treat infestation if the patient at once returns to work in an infected paddy-field. Treatment consists of a single dose of praziquantel which may be repeated after 1 month. Surgical resection of polypi and ulcers may be necessary, and the squamous cell cancer may require cystectomy. Obstruction, dilatation and stone formation in the ureters may require appropriate surgery.

Chapter 16

Bladder cancer

Bladder cancer

Because the bladder is lined by urothelium its neoplasms are nearly always transitional cell carcinomas, but if urothelium undergoes metaplasia into squamous or glandular epithelium (as happens with prolonged irritation or infection) then squamous cell cancer and adenocarcinoma can occur. Secondary cancer is sometimes seen from direct invasion from a primary tumour in the colon, rectum or uterus.

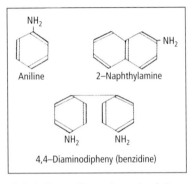

Figure 16.1 Aniline and its carcinogenic relatives.

Cancer of the urothelium

Aetiology

In 1894, Rehn noticed that workers in the aniline dye industry were developing an unduly large number of cancers of the bladder. Hueper subsequently showed that the cause was neither aniline, nor the finished dyestuffs, but a group of intermediate nitrophenols (Fig. 16.1) of which the most dangerous were β-naphthylamine and benzidine. These substances were also present in tobacco smoke and other industries including rubber moulding and the coal gas industry. All these industries have now eliminated these chemicals from their factories, but tobacco smoking continues to be the major hazard. In other parts of the world the prolonged irritation of the urothelium by schistosomiasis continues to be a major cause, probably added to by tobacco smoking.

Pathology

Bladder tumours are transitional cell cancers, but transitional epithelium (urothelium) can undergo metaplasia into either squamous epithelium or something which resembles glandular epithelium of the bowel. Bladder tumours may be single or multiple, and like all cancers, can take the shape of a cauliflower, an ulcer or a solid lump (Fig. 16.2). Truly benign papillomas are exceedingly rare, and

Lecture Notes: Urology, 6th edition. By John Blandy and Amir Kaisary. Published 2009 by Blackwell Publishing. ISBN: 978-1-4051-2270-2.

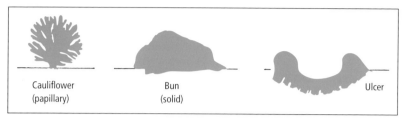

Figure 16.2 Macroscopic features of bladder cancer.

it is a pity that the term is often misused for the papillary forms of cancer. There are three grades of malignancy: G1, G2 and G3; G3 being the worst (Fig. 16.3).

Squamous carcinoma

Squamous changes are often seen in patches in G3 transitional cell cancers, and carry a bad prognosis. Pure squamous cancers arise in areas of squamous metaplasia and occur from the irritation of a stone, or in schistosomiasis: they have a thick layer of white keratin over them.

Adenocarcinoma

The glandular metaplasia seen in chronic infection and exstrophy may proceed to adenocarcinoma. Adenocarcinoma may also arise in the vestige of the foetal allantois, the urachus, as a cherry-like lump at the top of the bladder.

Spread of bladder cancer

Direct spread

Cancer may invade the surrounding fat and adjacent organs but never seems to cross Denonvilliers'

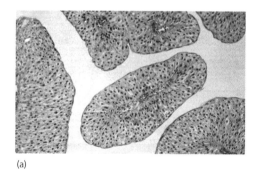

(a)

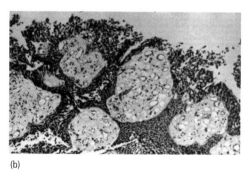

(b)

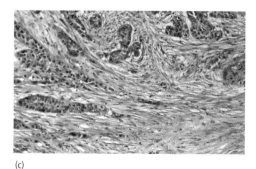

(c)

Figure 16.3 Grades of bladder cancer: (a) G1, (b) G2 and (c) G3.

fascia into the rectum, although cancer of the rectum appears to have no difficulty crossing into the bladder.

Implantation

Bladder cancer may be seeded into the urethra and possibly onto the opposite wall of the bladder – kiss cancer.

Lymphatic spread

Once a bladder cancer has invaded the detrusor muscle it finds there a rich plexus of lymphatics, and may spread into the nodes along the internal iliac artery and up along the aorta. There is also a direct connection between these lymphatics and the bone marrow of the pelvis, the upper end of the femur and the lower vertebrae.

Systemic spread

Metastases are occasionally seen in the lungs, liver or brain, but they are rare when compared with other cancers of the viscera.

Staging of bladder cancer

The International Union against Cancer uses the TNM system of staging, which is intended to enable different centres to compare their results (Fig. 16.4).

T staging system takes into account the evidence on which the depth of invasion has been assessed; e.g., the prefix **T** means a clinical guess, based on the assessment at the time of cystoscopy. A lower case **p** is added when there is a deep biopsy showing enough muscle to tell whether it has been invaded or not. An upper case **P** means that part or all of the bladder muscle has been removed.

N staging – the assessment of lymph node involvement – is always guesswork unless the lymph nodes have been removed surgically and sent for histological examination. Computed tomography (CT) and magnetic resonance imaging can detect the larger metastases with much less accuracy.

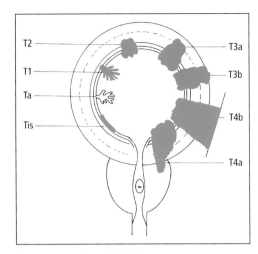

Figure 16.4 Staging of bladder cancer.

M staging – the detection of visceral metastases – depends on chest X-rays and ultrasound scanning of the liver.

The differences in the methods used to stage bladder cancer make it necessary to be wary of comparing the results of different forms of treatment, e.g. *total cystectomy* (where there is pathological evidence of depth of invasion and lymph node involvement) with *radiotherapy*, or *chemotherapy*, where staging based only on biopsies, CT and ultrasound scanning tends to underestimate the stage.

Clinical features

Screening of symptomless patients

Patients thought to be at risk, e.g. who worked in the chemical and rubber industry before the carcinogens were eliminated, have their urine screened annually for malignant cells. The cytological diagnosis of cancer depends on recognising large, multinucleated malignant cells in the urine (Fig. 16.5). If the tumour is G1 (well differentiated), the cells may go unrecognised unless by chance a broken-off frond of a papillary tumour is discovered. Automated *flow cytometry* measures the nuclear:cytoplasm ratio in large numbers of cells, thus avoiding observer error.

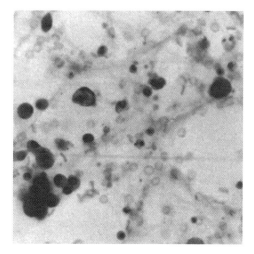

Figure 16.5 Malignant cells in the urine.

Symptoms

More than 80% of patients with bladder cancer present with haematuria (Fig. 16.6), which is the reason why every patient with haematuria must be cystoscoped. This rule applies whether the blood has been seen with the naked eye, or found by the stix test. The other 20% have *not* noticed blood in their urine and it is important to be aware of the other symptoms that should raise suspicion.

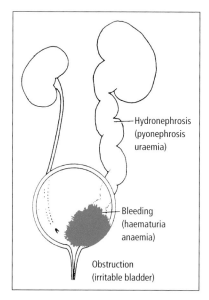

Figure 16.6 Clinical features of bladder cancer.

'Cystitis' with sterile pyuria: The urothelium around a bladder tumour is often inflamed, and the patient may have frequency and pain on voiding, just like bacterial ordinary cystitis. The clue is to find many 'pus cells' in the urine on microscopy, but no microorganisms in culture. Cancer cells can look very like leucocytes on ordinary microscopy. Sterile pyuria equals cancer until proven otherwise.

The decoy prostate: Most bladder cancers occur in elderly men, in whom irritability of the bladder often suggests prostatic outflow obstruction. To avoid this pitfall every man with 'prostatism' must have his urine tested for blood and cytology, and before prostatectomy the bladder must always be carefully examined by cytoscopy to rule out a small cancer.

Anaemia: Continued loss of blood in the urine sometimes brings a patient to the doctor with anaemia, out of all proportion to the size of the cancer.

Urinary infection: Infection occurring for no obvious reason in an elderly patient, particularly a heavy smoker, should be regarded with suspicion: it may be arising in the necrotic superficial part of a solid tumour.

Pain: This usually means that the cancer has invaded outside the bladder.

Physical signs

There are usually none, except in the rare tumour that arises from the urachus, when a hard mass is felt between the symphysis and the umbilicus. Otherwise if a mass can be felt, it signifies gross extension of the cancer.

Investigations

Doctors should respond to the finding of haematuria almost with a knee-jerk: haematuria = intravenous urogram (IVU) + cystoscopy.

The IVU
It may show a filling defect in the bladder (Fig.16.7), if a ureter is obstructed, it usually means

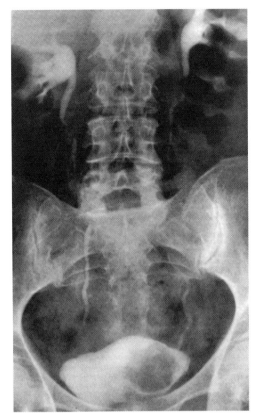

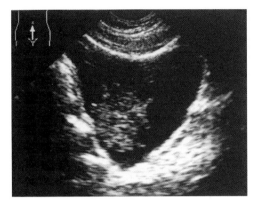

Figure **16.8** Ultrasound image showing bladder tumour.

tained with the resectoscope or cup forceps (Fig. 16.9). An adequate biopsy must include muscle from the base of the tumour to establish its depth of invasion (Fig. 16.10). After the tumour has been resected, bimanual examination is performed to detect induration which might signify deep muscle invasion, e.g. T3.

Treatment of bladder cancer

Figure **16.7** IVU in bladder cancer showing large filling defect.

Carcinoma in situ (G3 pTis)

This usually presents as 'cystitis' in a heavy smoker, who has seldom noticed haematuria. The urine is sterile on culture but full of cells which may be mistaken as leukocytes but prove to be malignant on cytological examination (Fig. 16.11). On cystoscopy the bladder may look a little inflamed. Biopsies of the urothelium confirm the diagnosis. The condition often responds with instillations of

the muscle near the ureteric orifice is invaded by tumour (T2).

Ultrasound

Scanning of the bladder may show a large tumour (Fig. 16.8) and can also indicate if there is obstruction of the ureters.

Cystoscopy

Flexible cystoscopy is quick and painless and does not require admission to hospital, but if a cancer has already been detected in the IVU the flexible cystoscopy can be bypassed and arrangements made for cystoscopy under general or regional anaesthesia.

Under anaesthesia the tumour is resected with the resectoscope, or at the very least a biopsy is ob-

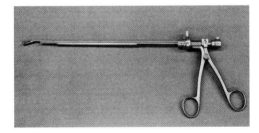

Figure **16.9** Storz cup biopsy forceps.

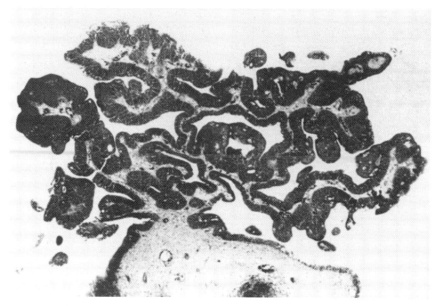

Figure 16.10 Biopsy taken with cup forceps.

bacille Calmette–Guérin (BCG) but must be kept under close review because it very easily turns into G3 invasive cancer.

Ta and T1 urothelial cancer

These tumours are initially removed by the resectoscope (Fig.16.12) at the time of the initial assessment. If two or three have been resected with an adequate base of muscle (Fig.16.13), the remainder may be coagulated with the diathermy ball (Fig.16.14). The same coagulation can be obtained using the neodymium–yttrium/aluminium/garnet

(YAG) laser (Fig.16.15). Patients are all carefully followed up at regular intervals by cytology and flexible cystoscopy. Recurrences are treated by transurethral resection or coagulation.

Transurethral resection of a bladder tumour

If the IVU or flexible cystoscopy has revealed a bulky tumour, serum should be sent for grouping in case blood is needed. The operation requires general or spinal anaesthetic, and can be prolonged and often quite difficult. The object is to

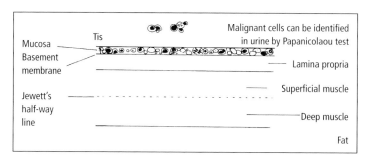

Figure 16.11 Flat carcinoma in situ.

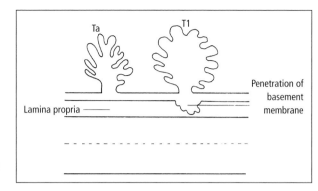

Figure 16.12 Ta and T1 carcinoma of the bladder.

cut away the 'bush' to reveal the 'stalk' of the cancer (Fig. 16.16). This is thoroughly coagulated to control bleeding, and then removed down to the deeper layers of the detrusor muscle. The 'bush' and the 'stalk' are sent separately to the laboratory so that the pathologist can tell how deeply the muscle is invaded. After all the bleeding has been stopped, a catheter is left in for a day or two. Possible complications include perforation of the wall of the bladder, absorption of irrigating fluid and bleeding.

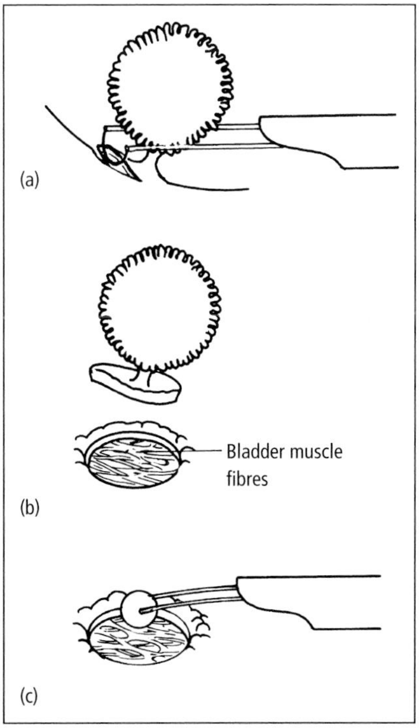

Adjuvant treatment

When there are very frequent and multiple recurrences the patient is given a course of intravesical instillations of BCG or some other antimitotic agent such as *Mitomycin*, *Adriamycin* or *Epodyl*. The most useful of these is BCG, but it causes a more or less painful cystitis. Although the response to the first course of BCG may be permanent, several maintenance courses are usually needed. Occasionally, the mild form of tuberculosis caused by the attenuated BCG may be followed by hepatitis, and require systemic antituberculous therapy. Instillation of a single dose of Mitomycin following the resection is often given to reduce the chance of recurrences.

Mitomycin treatment may cause an allergic reaction if it gets into contact with skin.

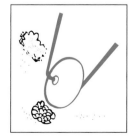

Figure 16.13 Small papillary tumour removed with resectoscope loop.

Figure 16.14 Small papillary tumour coagulated with rolyball electrode.

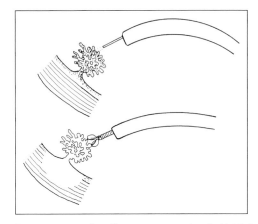

Figure 16.15 Small papillary tumour coagulated with YAG laser through flexible cystoscope.

G3 superficial cancers

Notable exceptions to this rather conservative policy are the uncommon G3 superficial papillary tumours. These carry such a bad prognosis that they are generally treated as if they are already invading the wall of the bladder (see below).

T2 and T3 invasive cancers

Most of these invasive cancers are G3. The distinction between T2 and T3 is somewhat artifi-

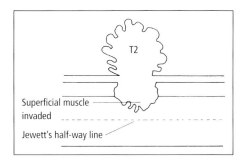

Figure 16.17 T2 bladder cancer.

cial, being based on an imaginary half-way line in the bladder muscle (Fig. 16.17). and (Fig. 16.18). Although the T2 cancers have a slightly better prognosis than T3, the difference is slight when compared with the dramatic worsening in survival once muscle begins to be invaded.

There are three main methods of treatment but there is no agreement as to how best to combine them.

Radiotherapy

About half of the G3 muscle-invading cancers will disappear completely after a course of 5500cGy from the linear accelerator. There is at present no way of predicting which cancer will respond, although the presence of squamous metaplasia and

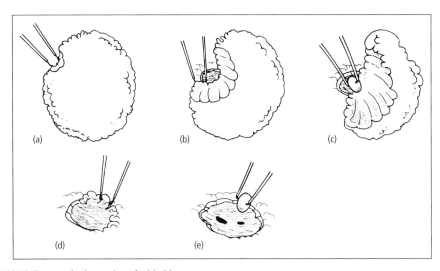

Figure 16.16 Transurethral resection of a bladder tumour.

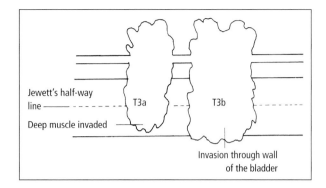

Figure 16.18 T3 bladder cancers.

staining for β-human chorionic gonadotrophin in the tissue strongly suggest that it will not.

Whether radiotherapy is chosen as the primary treatment or cystectomy, patients are followed up regularly for recurrences. If radiotherapy is chosen, 'salvage' cystectomy can be offered when the cancer fails to go away completely or comes back later. The disadvantages of radiotherapy are that if cystectomy is needed later on because of persistent or recurrent cancer, it is more difficult because radiation impairs healing. For the same reason it is more difficult to construct a new bladder from bowel, and the patient usually requires an ileal loop diversion. There may be also late complications from stricture in the bowel due to irradiation. The disadvantage of performing cystectomy as the method of first choice is that it denies the patient the pos-

sible adjuvant effect of radiation, and the chance of escaping cystectomy altogether. The long-term results are much the same and it is usual nowadays to explain the pros and cons of each method to the patient. Neo-adjuvant chemotherapy given before radiotherapy in three cycles over a 3- to 4-month period may improve the results.

Radical cystectomy

The operation has the advantage of giving a true P staging, and can be combined with removal of pelvic lymph nodes which may not only provide

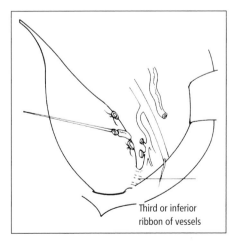

Figure 16.19 Dividing the main vessels of the bladder.

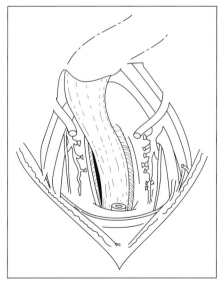

Figure 16.20 The empty pelvis after the bladder has been removed.

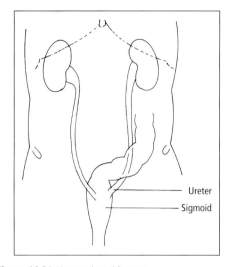

Figure 16.21 Ureterosigmoidostomy.

an accurate N staging, but may be curative. This is still a very major operation, and the patient needs to understand fully its grave implications. Nearly every male is rendered impotent although it is sometimes possible to protect the nerve supply to the penis and preserve potency. It is essential to discuss all the implications and problems that are associated with various forms of urinary diversion or the reconstruction of a new bladder from small or large bowel.

Preparation
The bowel is prepared with a high fluid intake and antibiotics. Anaemia is corrected by appropriate transfusion. Smoking is forbidden to min-imise chest infection. Six units of blood are cross-matched. The site for the ileal conduit is carefully selected and marked, using a dummy bag containing water.

Operative steps
All the lymph nodes are dissected off the aorta, common and internal iliac vessels on each side and sent for frozen section. If they are involved, the operation may be abandoned subject to the surgeon's choice. All the vessels supplying the bladder from the internal iliac artery are divided between ligatures, one after the other (Fig. 16.19). The ureters are divided about 5 cm away from the bladder (Fig. 16.20). When there are multiple tumours, there is a chance of recurrent cancer in the urethra so it is removed *en bloc* with the bladder and prostate.

Urinary diversion
Ureterosigmoidoscopy
This is the oldest technique. The ureters are led through tunnels in the wall of the sigmoid to prevent faeces from refluxing up them to the kidney (Fig. 16.21). Unfortunately, this operation was frequently followed by infection, and absorption of urine from the colon led to hyperchloraemic acidosis and renal failure. It has been almost entirely abandoned.

Ileal conduit
The ureters are anastomosed to one end of an isolated loop of ileum whose other end is led onto

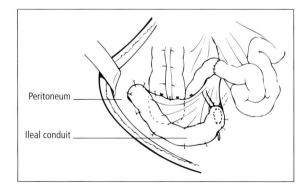

Figure 16.22 Ileal conduit.

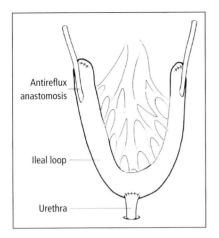

Figure 16.23 Neocystoplasty by Camey's method.

the skin to form a urostomy which is fitted with an adhesive bag (Fig. 16.22). Care must be taken in choosing the site for the stoma: it must not rub against the belt or lie in a scar or crease or else the bag will come unstuck.

Continent reservoir

After removing the bladder, a new one is constructed out of intestine. Numerous different methods are in use, but they all share certain principles: the bowel is open and closed in such a way that powerful peristaltic waves do not generate an increase in pressure, and precautions are taken to prevent reflux of urine from the new bladder up the ureters (Fig. 16.23).

If the urethra has been removed, a stoma is made onto the skin which is designed to be continent, so that the patient empties it from time to time with a catheter (Fig. 16.24).

If the urethra has not been removed, the reservoir can be sewn onto the stump of urethra and in many cases normal voiding is established (Fig. 16.25).

Absorption of urine from the bowel that has been used to make the new bladder still leads to the biochemical complication of hyperchloraemic acidosis, and these patients all need to be carefully followed to make sure that infection and stone

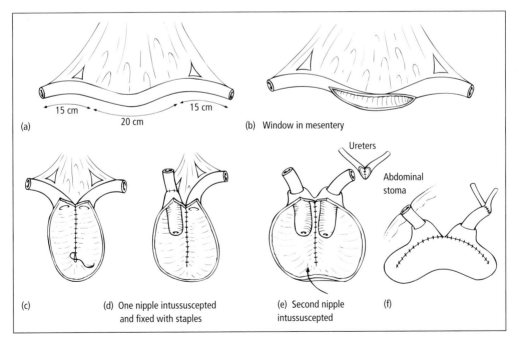

Figure 16.24 Kock's continent pouch.

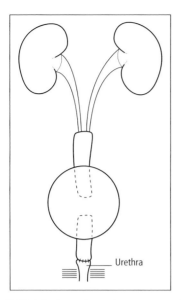

Figure 16.25 A Kock pouch may be anastomosed to the urethra.

formation in the new reservoir are detected and treated.

In Egypt, where cystectomy is required for squamous cell cancer after schistosomiasis, and the poor farm labourers cannot afford adhesive appliances, an ingenious method of diversion has been devised that makes use of the anal sphincter for continence (Fig. 16.26).

Complications of cystectomy

Ileus is always prolonged after cystectomy, the more so if there has been irradiation. During this time the bowel is kept deflated with a nasogastric tube or gastrostomy. Parenteral nutrition is given.

Leakage from the anastomoses between the ureters and the new bladder or ileal conduit, or from the reconstructed bladder, calls for strict vigilance in the early postoperative period. It is not unusual to have to revise the reservoir.

Pulmonary infection may require physiotherapy and antibiotics.

Deep venous thrombosis and pulmonary embolism are common complications and call for the usual prevention.

As with other urological operative procedures where minimally invasive surgical treatment is considered, laparoscopic cystectomy is being performed in suitably selected patients. It promises minimal blood loss, reduced length of ileus and quicker recovery.

Carcinoma of the urachus

This is very uncommon. The tumour is found on cystoscopy as a cherry-like swelling at the top of the bladder. Outside it is a much larger mass (Fig. 16.27). Biopsy shows adenocarcinoma. It is treated by a wide excision that takes all the

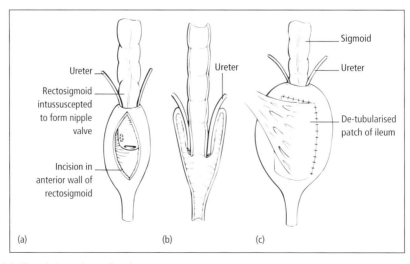

Figure 16.26 Ghoneim's continent diversion.

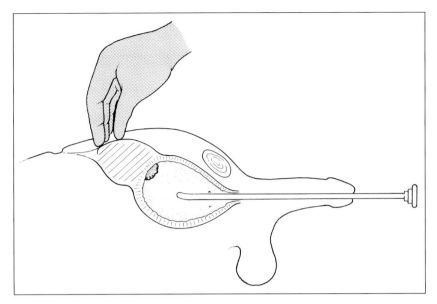

Figure 16.27 Carcinoma of the urachus.

triangle of tissue from the umbilicus down to the upper part of the bladder as well as all the regional lymph nodes. The small residual bladder is closed, but enlarges to its former capacity within a few weeks (Fig. 16.28).

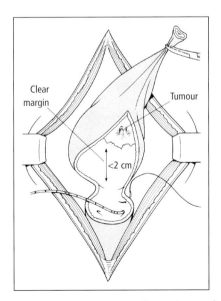

Clear margin

Tumour

<2 cm

Figure 16.28 Subtotal cystectomy for carcinoma of the urachus.

Combination chemotherapy

Various combinations of chemotherapeutic agents have been used which may give 'complete remission' in about half of the cases, but the treatments are all toxic and the response seldom prolonged. In most centres these regimes are reserved for patients who refuse or are not fit to undergo cystectomy, or as part of a combination with radiotherapy and 'salvage' cystectomy.

Palliation

When treatment has failed we are faced with an elderly patient, who has to void blood-stained urine with pain and difficulty every few minutes by day and night. Pain and infection in recurrent necrotic tumour makes the patient even more ill. Cancer of the bladder seldom brings a quick and merciful end from metastases.

Surgeons can do much towards the relief of suffering. A palliative urinary diversion with a ureterosigmoidostomy or an ileal conduit may stop the painful frequency. Palliative radiotherapy may stop bleeding and control pain. Pain-relieving medication should be provided at the control of the patient, i.e. when needed, not according to the hour, for pain knows no clock.

In the end, you are the doctor. You may be embarrassed and reluctant to visit your patients because you are ashamed of having so little to offer. Do not be mistaken: you can provide something of special value merely by being there from time to time. You can at least show that you are still the patient's friend, and that you care.

Chapter 17

The bladder: disorders of micturition

Diuresis

Polydipsia

Some patients, who are otherwise perfectly normal, form the habit of drinking an excessive amount of fluid: what goes in must come out. The diagnosis is made by asking the patient to keep a diary of his or her input and output of fluid.

Diabetes mellitus

Nothing is simpler than to test for glucose in the urine.

Diabetes insipidus

The anterior pituitary may fail to secrete antidiuretic hormone so that the patient is unable to concentrate urine. In children the enormous output of urine may lead to dilatation of the entire urinary tract. It can be treated with small doses of desmopressin.

Renal tubular disorders

The renal tubules fail to concentrate urine for three main reasons:

Lecture Notes: Urology, 6th edition. By John Blandy and Amir Kaisary. Published 2009 by Blackwell Publishing. ISBN: 978-1-4051-2270-2.

1 *Obstruction:* In bilateral hydronephrosis there is loss of the renal papillae so that water and salt are not reabsorbed. The urine is pale and of fixed specific gravity: the patient may become dehydrated and short of salt.

2 *Old age:* The pituitary fails to secrete the usual amount of antidiuretic hormone at night in old people, and at the same time the inferior vena cava fails to contract when the patient lies down, so that there is continued secretion of the atrial natriuretic hormone. Often this coexists with a mild degree of heart failure: the fluid retained in the lower limbs in the day as oedema is excreted at night. The diagnosis is easily made by asking the patient to keep a diary of the volumes of urine he or she passes at night. A small dose of desmopressin, e.g. 10–20 µg at bedtime, may give the patient a good night's rest.

3 *Sickle-cell disease:* Both homozygous and heterozygous forms of the disease may give rise to loss of function of the renal papillae. There is often microscopic haematuria; the urine has a fixed specific gravity and there is often a mild diuresis.

Neuropathy

Overstimulation of the afferent arm of the micturition reflex

Anything which makes the lining of the bladder more sensitive may provoke detrusor contraction

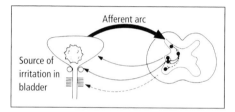

Figure 17.1 Overstimulation of the afferent arm of the micturition reflex.

before the bladder is full (Fig. 17.1), e.g. a stone, infection or carcinoma. At its worst the patient may be unable to inhibit this contraction and there is *urge incontinence*. Urodynamic studies will show uninhibited detrusor contractions, a normal flow rate, normal sphincters but a small voided volume.

Excessive central facilitation

Every examination candidate knows that anxiety can cause frequency (Fig. 17.2). In major anxiety states, frequency and even urge incontinence are common, and can make life intolerable. As a general rule this type of frequency only occurs in the daytime, in contrast to the frequency caused by irritation of the urothelium (above).

Lack of central inhibition of the reflex (Fig. 17.3)

Bed-wetting

Babies, like puppies and kittens, have to learn to inhibit the reflex emptying of the full bladder until

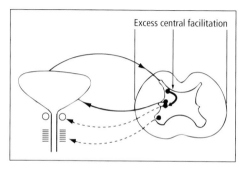

Figure 17.2 Excessive central facilitation.

time and place are convenient. In some children this learning process is delayed: many children who wet the bed seem to sleep unusually deeply. In practice it is difficult to know how far investigate an otherwise normal child, since bed-wetting is normal up to the age of 5 or 6. The urine should always be tested to exclude infection. Treatment exploits three principles:

1 A small dose of pituitary antidiuretic hormone is given (desmopressin 5–20 μg at bedtime).
2 Imipramine may work by lightening sleep, or by soothing the detrusor.
3 A buzzer which sounds when soaked with urine may establish a conditioned reflex provided the child is woken up and taken to the lavatory.

Senility

A humiliating feature of old age is incontinence of urine. A brief visit to a residential home for older people is enough to show how poorly we deal with it. There is usually a mixture of causes:
   lack of central inhibition, e.g. after a stroke;
   unawareness of a full bladder;
   detrusor instability; and
   immobility, from arthritis or weakness, preventing the person from getting to the lavatory on time.

The management is difficult and takes patience. A friendly reminder at regular intervals may encourage emptying of the bladder before there is an accident. Underpants with an absorbent pad placed outside a layer of unwettable material may keep the skin relatively dry, but the pads must be changed regularly, or they stink of ammonia. For men a condom urinal may keep him dry and comfortable (Fig. 17.4).

High spinal cord lesions

Messages from higher centres may be prevented from descending to S2 and S3 because of a lesion in the spinal cord. As a result there may be no coordination between contraction of the detrusor and relaxation of the sphincters. The detrusor contracts but the sphincters stay shut; the intravesical pressure rises and may cause dilatation of the ureters

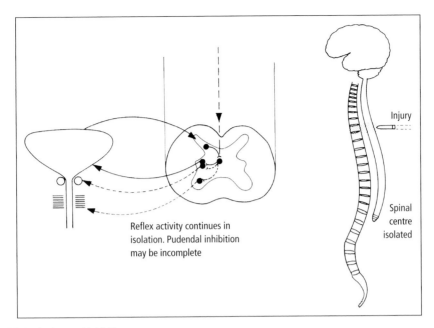

Figure 17.3 Lack of central inhibition.

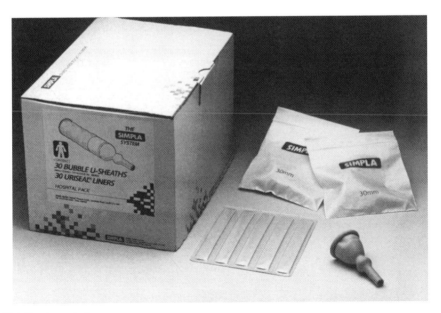

Figure 17.4 Condom urinal.

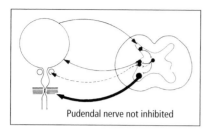

Figure 17.5 Failure of the external sphincter to relax when the detrusor contracts.

and obstructive uropathy (Fig. 17.5). The intravesical voiding pressure above which upper tract damage occurs is remarkably low, e.g. about 40 cm H_2O.

Trauma

When the spinal cord lesion is caused by trauma there is a period of *spinal shock* during which oedema makes the lesion seem worse than it really is. Hence at first no irreversible steps are taken, and the bladder is merely kept empty by regular intermittent catheterisation. When enough time has elapsed to allow the spinal shock to recover, *urodynamic* measurements may show that the sphincters are failing to relax in harmony with the contraction of the detrusor. There are now five possible options:

1 *Intermittent self-catheterisation:* The patient learns to pass a catheter regularly to keep the bladder empty. Unfortunately, with some high spinal cord lesions the detrusor may contract spontaneously even when the bladder is almost empty, so that the patient is wet, and a dangerously high pressure may be generated inside the bladder.

2 *Sphincterotomy:* The three parts of the sphincter in the male may be divided through a resectoscope one at a time, in the hope that the bladder will empty at a less than dangerously high pressure. Sometimes sphincterotomy of the bladder neck is enough to allow the patient to remain dry. More often it is necessary to divide the supramembranous and external sphincters as well.

3 *Clam cystoplasty:* When there is a very high pressure inside the bladder, it is opened like a clam, and a length of ileum is isolated, slit open and

sewn into the gap (Fig. 17.6). When the detrusor contracts, the patch of bowel balloons out and the pressure does not rise. This protects the kidneys. In some cases, with the assistance of a partial sphincterotomy, continence can be preserved. In others, the patient may still have to empty the bladder by intermittent clean self-catheterisation.

4 *Nerve root division and stimulation:* The afferent nerve roots to S2 and S3 may be divided, and the efferent nerve roots may be fitted with stimulators that enable the bladder to contract at will. These new procedures are undergoing trial and development (Fig. 17.7).

5 *Diversion:* Unfortunately many patients, particularly those with weakness of the upper limbs, or who are confined to a wheelchair, are not able to practice intermittent clean self-catheterisation. For them an ileal conduit or a form of continent diversion may be the most appropriate solution.

Lesions of the bladder centre at S2 and S3

Destruction of S2 and S3

The S2 and S3 segments are situated in the conus medullaris at the tip of the spinal cord, just opposite the disc between T12 and L1 vertebrae which are most often injured in accidents. To show whether they are intact there are three useful tests (Fig. 17.8):

1 *The bulbospongiosus reflex:* Pinch the glans penis and feel for a contraction of the bulbospongiosus muscle (Fig. 17.9).

2 *Cystometrogram:* The return of detrusor contractions (which can be provoked with ice-cold water) means that the reflex arc must be intact.

3 *Electromyography of the levator ani:* When the S2 and S3 segments are destroyed there are no action potentials in the levator ani.

Management

Without a reflex arc to drive it, the bladder becomes an inert floppy bag which fills up and then starts to leak – overflow incontinence. It can

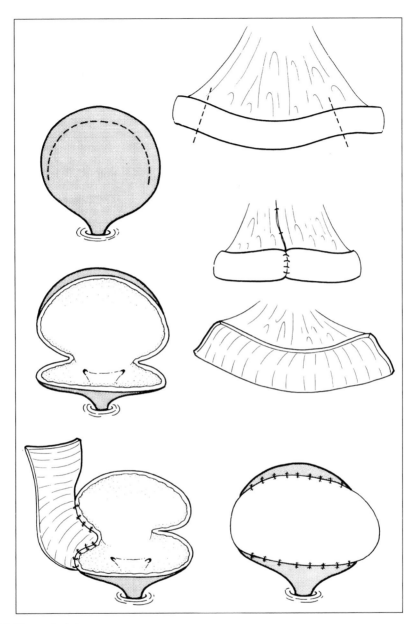

Figure 17.6 Clam cystoplasty.

sometimes be emptied by *suprapubic compression* although this may raise the pressure inside the bladder and threaten the upper tracts. Emptying may be incomplete and infection often develops in the residual urine. For these reasons patients are usually advised to perform intermittent clean self-catheterisation at least twice a day.

Irritation of S2 and S3

Cauda equina lesions
The most medial fibres of the cauda equina going to and from S2 and S3 may be irritated by a central prolapse of a lumbar intervertebral disc, causing a combination of frequency and impotence.

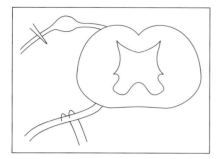

Figure 17.7 Nerve root division and stimulation.

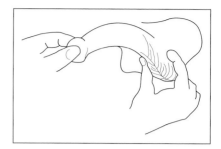

Figure 17.9 Bulbospongiosus reflex.

Removal of the offending disc may cure both disorders (Fig. 17.10).

Lesions of the pelvic autonomic nerves

Parasympathetic nerves

The pelvic parasympathetic nerves may be torn in *fractures* of the pelvis or removed in the course of *radical surgery* for cancer. Their *myelin sheaths* are frequently involved in *diabetes mellitus* and the *Shy–Drager* syndrome. The result is a big floppy bladder with an inert detrusor.

Sympathetic nerves

If the presacral sympathetic nerves are affected by these conditions the seminal vesicles and bladder neck do not contract during ejaculation with the result that there is retrograde emission of semen. The detrusor function is unaffected.

Detrusor instability

When no cause can be found for uninhibited contractions of the detrusor, it is called *detrusor instability*, so it is a diagnosis that can be made only by exclusion. A degree of detrusor instability is found in many normal people if subjected to careful urodynamic studies. Such detrusor contractions can be precipitated by coughing or straining, and can easily be confused with stress incontinence (see below). At present

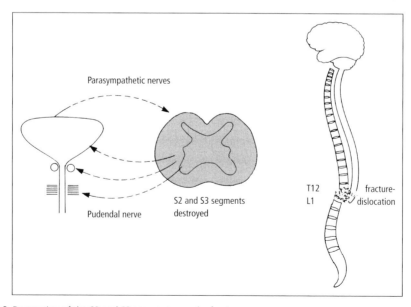

Figure 17.8 Destruction of the S2 and S3 segments, e.g. by fracture.

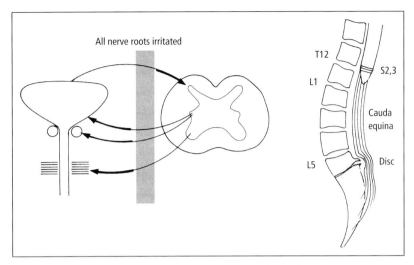

Figure 17.10 Cauda equina lesion irritating afferent and efferent limbs of the reflex arc.

the cause of detrusor instability is not known, with the result that there are many theories and many types of treatment, none of which are very effective.

Mechanical lesions of the bladder outlet

Obstruction

Whether the cause is neuropathic failure of the sphincters to relax in harmony with the contraction of the detrusor, obstruction by enlargement of the prostate, or a stricture of the urethra, there are two phases to the response of the detrusor:

1 *Compensatory hypertrophy:* The detrusor responds to the demand for a stronger contraction by an increase in the size and strength of its smooth muscle fibres, and a coarsening of the network in which they are arranged – trabeculation (Fig. 17.11). The urothelium begins to bulge out through the gaps in the network forming saccules which eventually balloon right outside the bladder as diverticula. During this phase of compensatory hypertrophy unstable detrusor contractions occur, generating a high pressure, and sometimes leading to incontinence of urine. This is one form of instability which can be reversed by removing the cause of the obstruction.

2 *Detrusor failure:* Like any muscle that has to go on working against abnormal resistance, the detrusor eventually gives up. Instead of emptying the bladder completely, it slowly permits the quantity of residual urine to increase. The time comes when detrusor contractions disappear entirely from the cystometrogram, perhaps because any weak end efforts of the muscle are absorbed by the thin-walled *diverticula*. The flow is reduced to a trickle, and then only the pressure in the bladder is increased by abdominal straining or coughing. Before long the huge floppy bladder dribbles without control – *retention with overflow* (Fig. 17.12). Such a bladder never recovers its normal function even with prolonged drainage and removal of the obstruction. The residual urine easily becomes infected. Stones or cancer may develop silently in the diverticula.

Detrusor–sphincter dyssynergia

Detrusor contraction without synchronous relaxation of the sphincters is easily understood when there is an obvious neurological disorder, but it may occur from time to time in otherwise normal people. Urodynamic studies show a high detrusor pressure, but one or other part of the sphincter fails to relax.

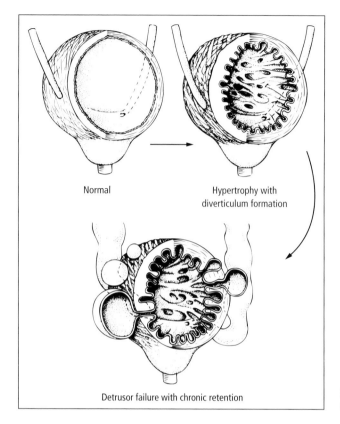

Normal

Hypertrophy with
diverticulum formation

Detrusor failure with chronic retention

Figure 17.11 Compensatory hypertrophy of the detrusor.

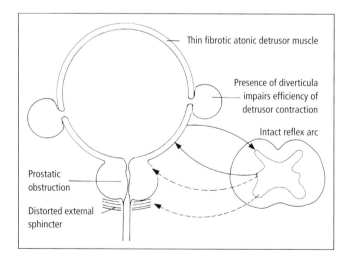

Thin fibrotic atonic detrusor muscle

Presence of diverticula impairs efficiency of detrusor contraction

Intact reflex arc

Prostatic obstruction

Distorted external sphincter

Figure 17.12 Detrusor failure.

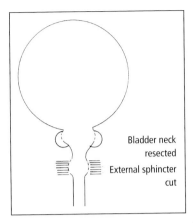

Figure 17.13 Incontinence following division of both sphincters.

The most common form is seen in middle-aged men, where the alpha-adrenergic fibres of the *bladder neck* fail to relax. This can be successfully treated with alpha-blockers such as *prazosin, indoramin or tamsulosin*. If this gives a good clinical result, the fibres may be divided by transurethral incision of the bladder neck.

When it is the *striated muscle* component of the sphincter that fails to relax, the diagnosis can be confirmed by electromyography of the levator ani muscle, which will show the action potentials continuing loudly when there ought to be electrical silence. Sometimes listening to the noise of the action potentials on a loudspeaker enables the patient to inhibit them herself – so-called biofeedback.

Sphincter damage

Prostatectomy: The bladder neck is removed as a deliberate part of the operation of transurethral resection for benign enlargement of the prostate and radical prostatectomy for cancer. Sometimes the supramembranous component of the external sphincter is cut by accident during transurethral resection (Fig. 17.13).

Fractured pelvis: The sphincters may be injured if the bladder neck is lacerated by a fracture of the pelvis, or if the fracture ruptures the presacral sympathetic nerves.

Cancer of the prostate: Prostatic cancer may infiltrate the sphincters causing them to lie permanently stiff and half-open.

Investigation

Urodynamic measurements show a normal, stable detrusor, but negligible outflow resistance.

Treatment

When the lesion is minor, the external sphincter may be strengthened by pelvic floor exercises. In more serious cases an appliance is used to compress the urethra.

The oldest is the *Cunningham clip* (Fig. 17.14), whose sponge–rubber jaws gently compress the urethra. It can be put on and off by the patient, is cheap and relatively safe but risks pressure injury to the urethra.

The newest is the Brantley–Scott artificial sphincter. A thin silicone balloon-shaped like a doughnut is placed round the urethra and connected to a reservoir which can be emptied or filled by a bulb placed under the skin where the patient can compress it. These expensive miracles of engineering are apt to suffer mechanical failure, infection and erosion into the urethra (Fig. 17.15).

Herniation of the base of the bladder through the pelvic floor

In women there is a short length of urethra above the levator ani shelf. When she coughs, the abdominal pressure squeezes this length of urethra

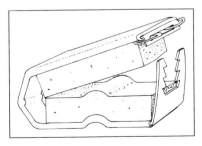

Figure 17.14 Cunningham clamp.

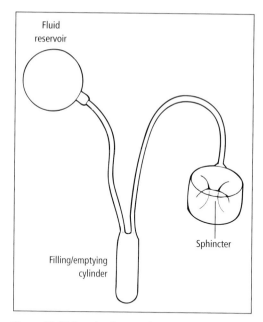

Figure 17.15 Brantley–Scott artificial sphincter.

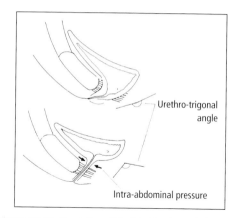

Figure 17.16 Herniation of the bladder through the pelvic floor: the aim of all operations is to lift the urethra up again so that any increase of intra-abdominal pressure will compress the urethra.

by exactly the same amount as it squeezes the bladder. In many women, especially (but not always) those who have borne children, the normal gap in the levator ani for the urethra is enlarged, and allows it to descend so that the intra-abdominal pressure can no longer squeeze it shut (Fig. 17.16). Now when the patient coughs or laughs there is a little spurt of urine – *stress incontinence*.

Diagnosis

Clinical examination

In genuine stress incontinence (GSI) there is leakage of urine when the patient coughs. This can be prevented by lifting up the anterior wall of the vagina with a finger on either side of the urethra (Bonney's or Marshall's test). The test should be done with the patient standing upright (Fig. 17.17).

Urodynamics

Because a similar escape of urine is seen in *detrusor instability* these patients need urodynamic testing

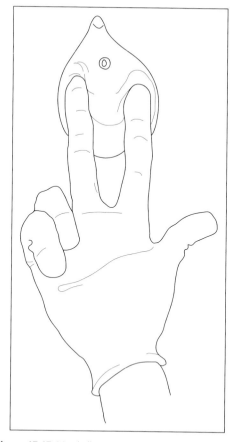

Figure 17.17 Marshall's test.

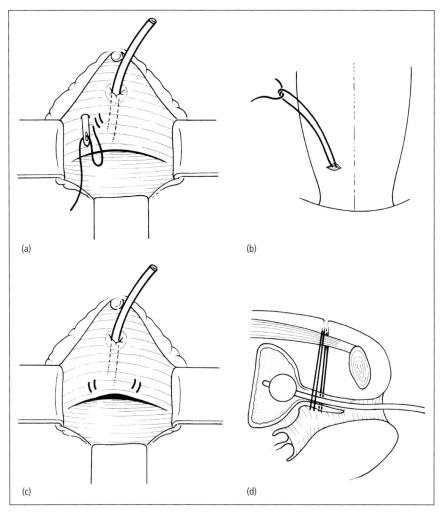

Figure 17.18 Stamey sutures.

to rule it out before they are accepted as having GSI.

Treatment of GSI

There are five procedures as follows:

1 *Stamey, Raz, Pereira sutures:* Described by various surgeons, non-absorbable sutures are placed to lift up the vaginal wall on either side of the urethra, just as in the Bonney–Marshall clinical test (Fig. 17.18). The operation is easy for the patient, but the stitches tend to cut out like cheesewire and there is a high recurrence rate after 2 years.

2 *Anterior colporrhaphy:* Through a vaginal incision the connective tissue on either side of the urethra is approximated to support the neck of the bladder. The long-term results are discouraging (Fig. 17.19).

3 *Burch colposuspension:* This is the classical and most reliable procedure, which has been 'invented' by several surgeons. Essentially, stitches are placed into the vaginal wall on either side of the urethra, and then through the pectineal fascia (Burch). The end result is to achieve something comparable to the Marshall–Bonney test (Fig. 17.20).

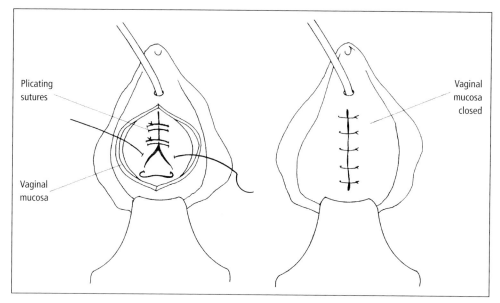

Figure 17.19 Anterior colporrhaphy.

4 *Sling operations:* A sling of some convenient material, preferably living rather than artificial, is used to lift up the bladder neck on a hammock. Millin used a strip of rectus abdominis fascia. Others use fascia or artificial materials, but these tend eventually to erode-like cheesewire into the bladder and form a stone (Fig. 17.21). New materials are continually being tried in the hope of improving the results of these sling operations.

5 *Periurethral injections:* Various substances have been injected around the bladder neck to give bulk to the tissue around the bladder neck and sphincter. A suspension of Teflon was the first, but was given up when it was discovered that the material got into the brain of experimental animals. Collagen paste and suspensions of the patient's own fat are now under trial (Fig. 17.22).

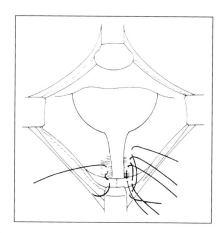

Figure 17.20 Vaginal colposuspension.

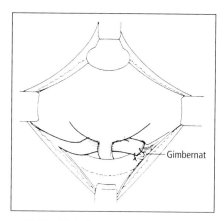

Figure 17.21 Millin's sling operation.

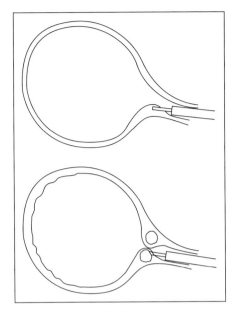

Figure 17.22 Injections of Teflon or collagen paste around the bladder neck.

Pharmacological treatment

Medication can be helpful in the common disorders of bladder function (Fig. 17.23). The smooth muscle of the detrusor is *cholinergic*. To encourage the bladder to empty, one can give bethanechol to release acetylcholine from

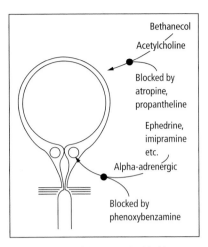

Figure 17.23 Action of drugs on the bladder.

the postganglionic fibres in the detrusor. To discourage an over-active bladder, one may try propantheline or one of the many medications which belong to the anticholinergic family and are claimed to have more efficacy and fewer adverse effects. The smooth muscles of the sphincters are alpha-adrenergic (Fig. 17.23). Weakness of the smooth muscle of the sphincters is occasionally helped by an adrenergic drug such as ephedrine or imipramine, and alpha-blockers are sometimes effective in treating detrusor sphincter dyssynergia.

Chapter 18

The prostate gland: benign disorders

Surgical anatomy

The prostate is made up of several zones which fit into each other like an egg in an egg-cup. Benign enlargement mainly arises in the transition zone, cancer in the peripheral zone. The ejaculatory ducts run between the two main zones and empty into the urethra at the verumontanum (Fig. 18.1).

The prostate is closely related to the three elements of the sphincter in the male:

The bladder neck (internal sphincteric mechanism) is a collection of alpha-adrenergic smooth muscle, supplied by sympathetic nerve fibres.

The supramembranous external sphincter, partly smooth muscle, partly striated, is just below the verumontanum, and also supplied by sympathetic nerve fibres.

The levator ani, voluntary striated muscle supplied by the pudendal nerve.

Anatomical relations

Anterior to the prostate is the symphysis pubis. Posteriorly, the prostate is separated from the rec-

Lecture Notes: Urology, 6th edition. By John Blandy and Amir Kaisary. Published 2009 by Blackwell Publishing. ISBN: 978-1-4051-2270-2.

tum by the fascia of Denonvilliers. Behind and above the prostate lie the bladder, seminal vesicles, vasa deferentia and ureters (Fig. 18.2).

Structure of the prostate

The prostate is made up of glandular tubules which open into the back of the urethra. Each tubule is emptied by a contractile sleeve of smooth muscle. Tubules and muscles are supported by stroma of connective tissue. The three elements of the prostate – glands, muscle and stroma – can all enlarge and shrink at different times of life (Fig. 18.3).

The prostate gland has a thin film of connective tissue which separates the surrounding fat and veins from the glandular tissue. This is important, because the 'capsule' is repeatedly referred to in discussions on the surgery of the prostate, nearly always incorrectly (Fig. 18.4). The anterior fibromuscular stroma is a thick sheet of connective tissue that covers the entire anterior surface of the prostate. The peripheral zone is the largest zone of the prostate. The central zone is a small region traversed by the ejaculatory ducts. The transition zone is a small group of ducts arising at a single point at the junction of the proximal and distal urethral segments.

In childhood there are very few glands: they appear and develop in puberty. In old age hypertrophy of one or all three elements in the

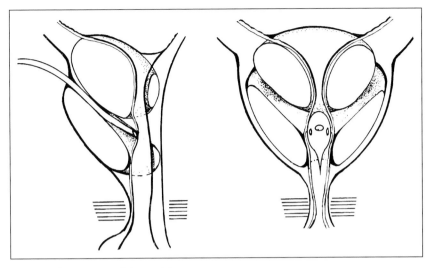

Figure 18.1 Inner and outer zones of the prostate.

transition zone around the periurethral area gives rise to the nodules of benign prostatic enlargement. These nodules vary in size and may compress the outer zone of the prostate into a thin shell and deform the prostate so as to give the appearance of having two 'lateral lobes' and one 'middle lobe'. These 'lobes' are not true functional entities, but artefacts caused by the way the prostate is confined by the symphysis and the bladder.

Physiology

The prostate is an accessory sex gland whose primary function is the support and promotion of male sperm function and fertility. During ejaculation it is thought that the prostate contracts to secrete about 0.5–1.0 mL of fluid which is added to the ejaculate. The acini of these ducts are composed of secretory cells, basal cells and neuroendocrine cells. It is the epithelial secretory cells

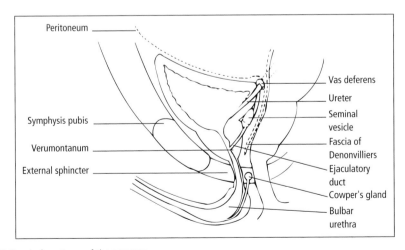

Figure 18.2 Surgical anatomy of the prostate.

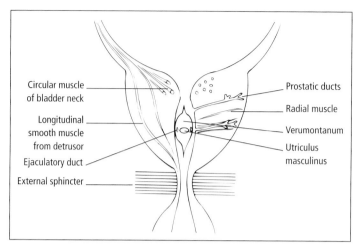

Figure 18.3 Structure of the prostate.

Circular muscle of bladder neck

Longitudinal smooth muscle from detrusor

Ejaculatory duct

External sphincter

Prostatic ducts

Radial muscle

Verumontanum

Utriculus masculinus

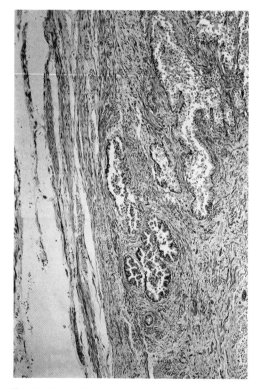

Figure 18.4 Section through the edge of the prostate showing how the connective tissue of the 'capsule' is continuous with that surrounding the vessels outside. (Courtesy of the late Mr Basil Page.)

that produce both prostate-specific antigen and prostate acid phosphatase.

Inflammation of the prostate

Prostatitis is overdiagnosed in patients with non-specific perineal discomfort or lower urinary tract symptoms. In 1995, classification of the prostatitis syndromes addressed the categories of the disease based on the patient history, physical examination and urine analysis/culture as the cornerstones (Table 18.1).

Acute prostatitis

Acute bacterial prostatitis is a febrile illness with sudden abrupt onset. There are marked genitourinary symptoms and often a positive bacterial urine culture.

Obstruction downstream to the prostate may force urine up into its ducts and if the urine is infected it causes inflammation. Blood-borne infection is equally common.

Whatever the route of the infection, the prostate becomes enlarged, painful on rectal palpation, and may cause painful and obstructed micturition. Pathogens may be recovered from the urine. Colour Doppler transrectal ultrasound scanning may show hyperaemia (Fig. 18.5).

Table 18.1 Classification of the prostatitis syndromes.

Category	Name	Definition
I	Acute bacterial	Acute infection of the prostate
II	Chronic bacterial	Chronic infection of the prostate
III	Chronic pelvic pain syndrome	Symptoms without evidence of infection
IV	Asymptomatic	Incidental inflammation (prostate biopsy)

National Institutes of Health Summary Statement, 1995.

Treatment

An antibiotic that can reach the alkaline milieu of the prostate is needed, e.g. trimethoprim, erythromycin or ciprofloxacillin. A good combination is a short course of ciprofloxacillin in the acute attack, followed by 4–6 weeks of a low dose of trimethoprim. In most cases acute prostatitis resolves completely. Very rarely there is suppuration and an abscess forms which is best drained transurethrally, before it bursts spontaneously into the rectum (Fig. 18.6). Acute prostatitis is a disorder which may relapse without warning.

Chronic prostatitis

Persistent discomfort in the perineum with painful micturition is often attributed to chronic prostatitis. To prove it, urine is collected for culture in two parts (VB1 and VB2). Then the prostate is massaged transrectally to express fluid, which is collected (EPS). Finally a third urine specimen is collected (VB3). A diagnosis of infection in the prostate is made if the colony count of bacteria in EPS and VB3 is more than in VB1 and VB2.

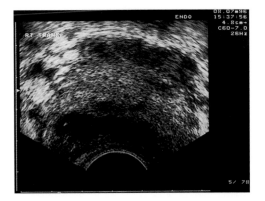

Figure 18.5 Transrectal Doppler scan showing hyperaemia in a case of acute prostatitis.

The organisms that are recovered may be the usual *Escherichia coli* but *Chlamydia trachomatis* and *Trichomonas vaginalis* are found from time to time. Their detection requires special culture techniques.

Investigations

Transrectal ultrasound with colour Doppler imaging will show hyperaemia.

Treatment

The principles of the treatment of chronic bacterial prostatitis are the same as for any persistent bacterial infection, with the added difficulty that in the prostate the milieu is alkaline and many of the standard antibiotics do not penetrate the gland. For Chlamydia, tetracyclines are usually effective. Trichomonas requires a week's course of metronidazole.

Non-bacterial prostatitis

An inflammatory syndrome is symptomatically indistinguishable from chronic bacterial prostatitis. It similarly presents with pyuria but no typical uropathogens are cultured in prostatic secretions and urine. Specialised cultures may grow Chlamydia, Candida, Cryptococcus, Mycobacterium or parasites (e.g. *T. vaginalis*).

Prostatodynia

For each patient who has proven bacterial infection, there are dozens who complain of vague pain in the perineum, discomfort on voiding and sexual inadequacy. Usually there is a psychosexual problem, made worse when they are told that their chronic prostatitis must be treated by a course of

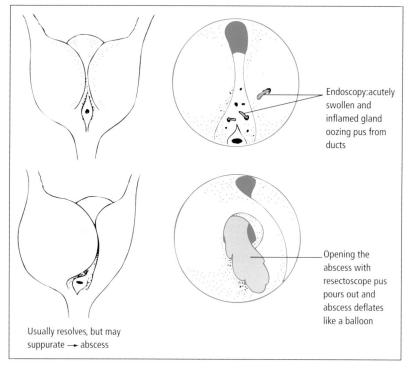

Endoscopy:acutely swollen and inflamed gland oozing pus from ducts

Opening the abscess with resectoscope pus pours out and abscess deflates like a balloon

Usually resolves, but may suppurate → abscess

Figure 18.6 Acute prostatitis usually resolves but may form an abscess.

'prostatic massage', a treatment which is as uncomfortable as it is irrational – no other inflammation is made better by being forcibly squeezed.

In the absence of any scientific explanation for it, the treatment is necessarily unsatisfactory. The important thing is not to make it worse by futile or meddlesome intervention. Sympathy and the provision of analgesia, e.g. with diclofenac suppositories, often brings about symptomatic relief. Inevitably patients with prostatodynia are treated with alpha-blocker medications, and sitz baths and given various herbal preparations for which the claims are seldom supported by any evidence.

Benign enlargement of the prostate

Aetiology

Over the age of 40, all men have some nodular hyperplasia in the transition zone of their prostate. The cause is not known although there is endless speculation as to some imbalance between oestrogens and androgens, based on animal experiments of doubtful relevance to humans. Only one in ten will ever develop obstruction that needs treatment. Size is irrelevant: the smallest prostates may cause severe obstruction; huge glands none at all. Constriction of the prostatic urethral lumen is the issue.

Pathology

Three factors act to cause obstruction as follows:
1 *Smooth muscle:* The alpha-adrenergic smooth muscle fibres in the prostate, especially around the bladder neck, fail to relax as the detrusor contracts. This may accompanied by hypertrophy of the smooth muscle (Fig. 18.7) and endoscopy may show a tight ring at the bladder neck without enlargement of the prostate.
2 *Adenoma:* A more or less large bulge of any or all three 'lobes' of the prostate may obstruct

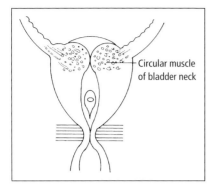

Figure 18.7 Hypertrophy of the smooth muscle of the bladder neck.

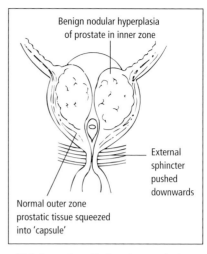

Figure 18.9 Formation of bulky adenomas in the prostate.

the lumen. The middle lobe alone may protrude like a thumb into the bladder (Fig. 18.8). As the inner zone of the prostate enlarges, the outer zone is compressed into a shell, often (incorrectly) called the 'capsule', while the verumontanum is displaced down towards the external sphincter (Fig. 18.9).

3 *Detrusor failure:* In the first phase the detrusor muscle fibres hypertrophy and become stronger and more jumpy. Later they become weaker and less forcible, and this weakness is often an additional factor contributing to the development of further obstruction. Detrusor failure may occur suddenly or gradually.

Sudden acute detrusor failure may be precipitated by some other unrelated illness, e.g. a heart attack or confinement to bed for an operation on some other system, and it causes acute retention of urine. This is very painful. The bladder is felt as a hard suprapubic mass. Often all that is necessary is to let the urine out with a catheter and normal voiding will be resumed.

In gradual chronic detrusor failure there is no pain. The big distended bladder is often soft and difficult to feel. A little urine escapes from time to time – overflow incontinence (Fig. 18.10). Among these men some develop a third, common condition: after a long crescendo of progressive obstruction, they suddenly cannot void at all. This is referred to as acute-on-chronic retention.

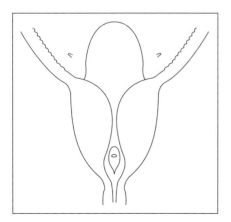

Figure 18.8 The middle 'lobe' may protrude into the bladder.

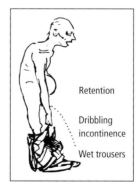

Figure 18.10 Overflow incontinence.

Complications of obstruction

1 *Changes in the detrusor:* If the obstruction is not relieved, the detrusor will develop trabeculation, sacculation and form diverticula. Eventually it loses the power to contract, which may be irreversible.

2 *Complications from residual urine:* Infection and stone formation are apt to occur whenever there is a large pocket of stagnant urine.

3 *Obstructive uropathy:* Neglected obstruction leads to loss of renal tubular function, the inability to conserve water or salt, and ultimately to impaired glomerular filtration leading to uraemia.

The objectives of the management of benign enlargement of the prostate are quite simple, to diagnose and relieve obstruction before any of these three complications occurred.

Diagnosis of prostatic obstruction

History

The symptoms that bring the patient to the doctor before the patient has developed complications are usually frequency of micturition and a poor flow, but these are not specific, and every patient requires a careful history. An attempt to quantify patients' symptoms was introduced by the American Urological Association Clinical Practice Guidelines (International Prostate Symptom Score – I-PSS) who suggest that it should be used by all primary care physicians who evaluate patients with benign prostate hypertrophy (Table 18.2). The questions cover both obstructive and irritative symptoms. Generally the patients are divided into patients with mild score (<7),

Table 18.2 International Prostate Symptom Score (I-PSS).

	Not at all	<1 in 5	<Half the time	About half the time	>Half the time	Almost always	Score
1 Incomplete emptying							
Sensation of not emptying the bladder completely after finishing urination	0	1	2	3	4	5	
2 Frequency							
You have to urinate again less than 2 hours after you finished urinating	0	1	2	3	4	5	
3 Intermittency							
Stop and start frequently when urinating	0	1	2	3	4	5	
4 Urgency							
Difficulty to postpone urinating	0	1	2	3	4	5	
5 Weak stream	0	1	2	3	4	5	
6 Straining							
You have to push or strain to begin urination	0	1	2	3	4	5	
7 Nocturia	0	1	2	3	4	5	
Total I-PSS =							

Quality of life due to urinary symptoms
How do you feel if you have to spend the rest of life with urinary function as it is now?

Delighted		Pleased	Satisfied	Mixed		Dissatisfied	Unhappy	Terrible
0		1	2	3		4	5	6

There are no standard recommendations in grading patients with mild, moderate or severe symptoms, but patients can be classified as follows: mild symptoms = 0–7, moderate symptoms = 8–19 or severe symptoms = 20–25 points.

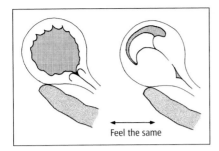

Figure 18.11 The finger in the rectum cannot distinguish urine under pressure in the bladder from a big prostate.

moderate (8 to 19) and severe (>20). It should never be a substitute for listening to the patient carefully, especially since these symptom scores do not match objective evidence of obstruction.

Physical signs

Abdominal palpation may reveal a chronically obstructed bladder but this is a late feature of the disease. Rectal examination cannot distinguish between a tight bladder full of residual urine and a large prostatic adenoma (Fig. 18.11), nor can it feel a middle lobe that sticks up into the bladder out of reach of the finger (Fig. 18.12).

Investigations

1 *Flow rate:* Flow rates vary from day to day, and a poor flow may not necessarily mean obstruction: it may result from a weak detrusor, while on the

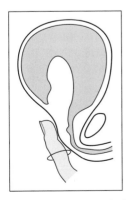

Figure 18.12 The rectal finger cannot feel a large middle lobe.

other hand if the detrusor has undergone considerable hypertrophy it can compensate for obstruction and produce a good flow rate. Nevertheless an impaired flow rate of <10 mL/s is a significant part of the clinical pattern (Fig. 18.13).

2 *Residual urine:* The residual urine can be measured by abdominal ultrasound. Again this may vary from day to day. The abdominal ultrasound may also detect dilatation of the ureters and renal pelves and will reveal gross trabeculation and diverticula (Fig. 18.14).

3 *Transrectal ultrasound:* The volume of the prostate can be measured from the ultrasound image, and may help in planning treatment. It may detect prostatic cancer (Fig. 18.15).

4 *Urodynamic studies:* The only way of making certain that there is outflow obstruction to the bladder is by means of a comprehensive urodynamic investigation which must include the measurement of the pressure inside the bladder during micturition. Since, to be accurate, this involves inserting urethral catheters and rarely a suprapubic one, these tests are only used when there is real doubt about the diagnosis, especially when the patient's main symptoms are frequency and urgency.

Differential diagnosis

1 *Cancer:* The symptoms of bladder cancer may so closely mimic prostatism that every elderly man complaining of frequency should have his urine examined for red cells and cancer cells.

2 *Stricture:* The symptoms of obstruction by enlargement of the prostate are identical to obstruction from a urethral stricture, so that if there is, for example, a history of previous catheterisation, e.g. during cardiac surgery or some other urethral instrumentation, the diagnosis of stricture should be considered.

3 *Neuropathy:* Neuropathic lesions, especially a central lumbar disc protrusion, can mimic prostatism.

4 *Polyuria:* The alteration in the excretion of the pituitary antidiuretic hormone that occurs in old age and in mild heart failure causes nocturnal urinary frequency which has nothing to do with the prostate.

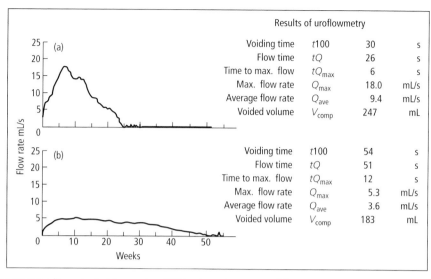

Results of uroflowmetry			
Voiding time	$t100$	30	s
Flow time	tQ	26	s
Time to max. flow	tQ_{max}	6	s
Max. flow rate	Q_{max}	18.0	mL/s
Average flow rate	Q_{ave}	9.4	mL/s
Voided volume	V_{comp}	247	mL
Voiding time	$t100$	54	s
Flow time	tQ	51	s
Time to max. flow	tQ_{max}	12	s
Max. flow rate	Q_{max}	5.3	mL/s
Average flow rate	Q_{ave}	3.6	mL/s
Voided volume	V_{comp}	183	mL

Figure 18.13 Urine flow rates in (a) normal and (b) benign enlargement of the prostate.

5 *Depression:* Many a sad old widower wakes in the small hours because he is lonely and depressed. He goes to the toilet, but cannot get back to sleep. So, he gets up and makes a cup of tea. Then he must urinate again, and so on. The patient will tell you the diagnosis if you only listen.

Treatment

1 *Wait and see:* Many elderly men go through a year or two during which their prostate irritates them, but not very severely, and then it gets better without any treatment (or if they are given a placebo in the course of a clinical trial). They may still have to urinate once or twice in the night, but their daytime activities are unaffected. They have a reasonable flow rate and their residual urine is negligible. The patient is advised to come back and report progress in 6 months or so.

2 *Drugs:*

(a) *Alpha-blockers:* When the prostate is small and the patient's symptoms dominated by

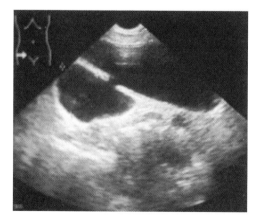

Figure 18.14 Ultrasound after trying to empty the bladder showing large residual as well as a diverticulum.

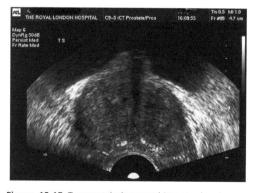

Figure 18.15 Transrectal ultrasound images showing enlargement of the prostate.

frequency, the problem may be a mild form of detrusor–sphincter dyssynergia and an alpha-blocker, e.g. Tamsulosin, often relieves symptoms. It is a tablet which aims at relaxing the circular muscle fibres around the bladder outlet (neck). It is taken at a dose of one tablet daily. The response to therapy is usually swift. It is a member of a family of medications that is commonly taken to reduce the elevated blood pressure. However, it does not necessarily lead to problems with patients receiving it to help with bladder emptying. Some patients might experience dizziness or a tendency to faint with sudden quick movements. These symptoms seem to settle down gradually in most patients. The tablet can have an impact in some patients with regards to sexual function. This takes the form of decreased ejaculate volume and some men might describe it as 'dry orgasm'.

(b) *5 Alpha-reductase inhibitor (Finasteride)*: This drug prevents a hydrogen atom being added to testosterone to activate it inside the prostate cell, and aims at shrinking the glandular part of the prostate. It makes the prostatic-specific antigen level fall, and in many patients appears to relieve symptoms. It is taken at a dose of one tablet at night for at least 3–6 months. Response to therapy can take up to 12 months in some cases, and unfortunately only 50% of patients will respond to treatment. There is no way of predicting who will and who will not respond. Those who do respond continue to receive tablets indefinitely. It occasionally has an effect on sexual function which includes: loss of potency (approximately 8%), decreased libido (approximately 5%) and decreased ejaculate volume (approximately 4%).

(c) The two drugs may be taken together in the first instance for a short period, usually for 3 months, to achieve a quick response following which a decision with regard to maintain one agent only is taken.

(d) *Phytotherapy*: These products are not the actual plants but are extracts derived from either the roots, the seeds, the bark or the fruits of the various plants used. Their mechanism of action is generally unknown. Examples include Saw Palmetto Berry (*Serenoa repens*), African Plum (*Pygeum africanum*), South African Star Grass (*Hypoxis rooperi*) and others.

3 *Surgery:*

Open prostatectomy: Around 1890, it was found almost by accident that the adenoma in the inner zone could be enucleated from the compressed shell of outer zone with a finger. In the early days this was performed via a suprapubic incision into the bladder, or through a perineal incision. In 1943, Millin developed the retropubic approach which is still used for very large glands (Fig. 18.16).

Transurethral resection: Improved technology made it possible to remove the inner zone adenoma with a telescope passed along the urethra (Fig. 18.17). This operation, which is usually performed under televisual control, carries an operative mortality of less than 1%, but there are still complications. Bleeding can be severe during the operation.

Stricture develops in the urethra afterwards in about 3% of men. Because the bladder neck is removed along with the prostate there is retrograde ejaculation of semen.

Impotence occurs in 10–15% after prostatectomy. Incontinence of urine may be the result of a technical mistake whereby the supramembranous external sphincter is injured, or may be due to persistent detrusor instability. It is one reason for being cautious in men who have frequency as their presenting feature.

4 *Transurethral incision of the prostate*: Instead of removing the inner zone, an incision is made through the bladder neck and prostate (see Fig. 18.18). There is less bleeding and a shorter hospital stay. No tissue is removed for histological diagnosis and the long-term results are still uncertain.

5 *Transurethral vaporisation of the prostate:* The prostatic tissue can be coagulated or vaporised by a special diathermy current or a laser (Fig. 18.19). The method appears to remove the inner zone tissue in a way that is comparable to transurethral resection but the long-term complication rate and results are still unknown.

183

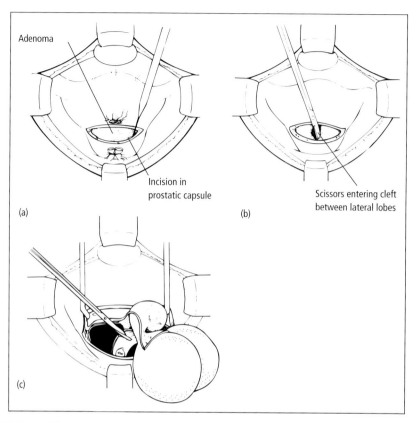

Figure 18.16 Retropubic prostatectomy.

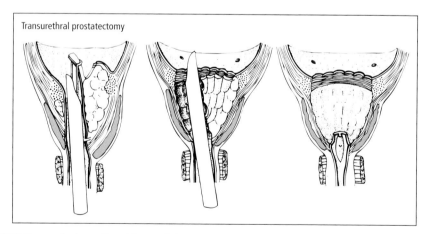

Figure 18.17 Transurethral resection of the prostate.

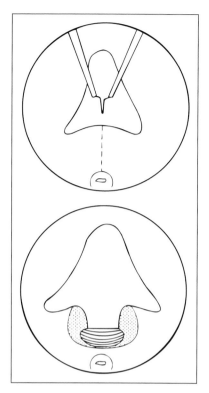

Figure 18.18 Transurethral incision of the prostate.

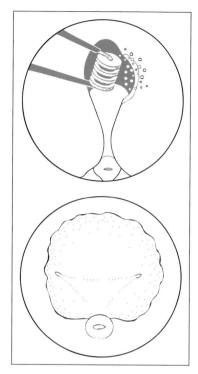

Figure 18.19 Transurethral vaporisation of the prostate using diathermy.

6 *Transurethral hyperthermia microwave therapy:* In this recent method, a beam of thermal energy emission from a urethral catheter targets the central part of the prostate gland (Fig. 18.20). It is focused to reach a high intensity in the target tissue where absorption of the energy heats and cooks the tissue at 42–44°C inducing cell death. A cooling balloon surrounds the probe to protect the urethral mucosa from the high temperature. Early results claim there may be some improvement in symptom scores in the I-PSS.

7 *Balloon dilatation:* A balloon is introduced in the prostatic urethra and inflated to a high pressure stretching the bladder neck and prostatic urethra. It is relatively a simple procedure but the results have been short lived and disappointing.

8 *Intraprostatic stents:* Insertion of a hollow tube within the prostatic urethra has been proposed as an alternative to long-term catheterisation in patients who are medically unfit for surgery. Several materials had been produced including spiral

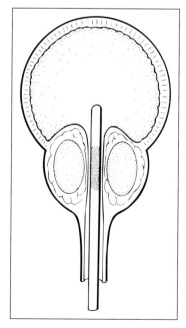

Figure 18.20 Transurethral hyperthermia of the prostate.

185

stainless steel, titanium mesh and biodegradable stents. Their use is associated with risks of encrustations, spontaneous displacement and tendency to long-term failure. Careful evaluation of long-term outcome is necessary.

Conclusion

More studies are needed to establish the long-term outcomes and complications of all these newer techniques in comparison to the conventional surgical prostatectomy. The choice should be discussed with the individual patient.

Practical management of retention disorders

• *Acute retention of urine*: When this follows some other illness, e.g. a recent heart attack or an operation to replace the hip, the bladder is emptied with a catheter which is left in position until the patient is up and about. When it occurs out of the blue, it is reasonable to see if the patient can empty his bladder – the so-called trial without catheter.
• *Acute-on-chronic retention*: When acute retention develops after a long crescendo of prostatic symptoms the catheter is left in, and arrangements are made for prostatectomy as soon as possible. The patient can safely go home during this interval wearing an indwelling catheter but he should be given a definite date, within a week or two, for his operation.
• *Chronic retention*: This is an entirely different entity because (i) the detrusor is often badly damaged, and (ii) there may be severe impairment of renal function with dehydration, salt-depletion and anaemia. If the creatinine is elevated one may be sure that the patient is also dehydrated, etc.

After the bladder is emptied, there may be a profuse post-obstructive diuresis during which such a large volume of fluid is lost that the patient may become shocked. Intravenous saline may be needed to make up the deficiency in extracellular volume. Fortunately the renal tubules usually recover, but during this time anaemia may require transfusion, heart failure may require treatment, and the mental condition of the patient may need care. The old man is sick, frightened, confused and

fuddled by medication. He needs kind voices to talk to, plenty of light, company and stimulation. The last things he needs are isolation and sedation. There is no company he needs so much as that of his family and friends. A little alcohol, within reason, may comfort him: it never did the kidneys any harm whatever it might have done to his liver.

As soon as his fluid balance is corrected and his creatinine is levelled off, his operation should be carried out. Such patients should not be submitted to a fruitless trial without catheter.

Preparations for prostatectomy

• *Consent: Whatever technique is used*, retrograde ejaculation is likely to occur and must be explained. The younger man who might still wish to have children might want to weigh this in the balance against the risks of putting off the removal of the obstruction. At any age the risks of ejaculatory impotence must be explained.
• *Blood loss:* After open or transurethral resection, loss of blood can be sudden, unpredictable and occasionally life-threatening. Blood should always be grouped and if the gland is known to be very large, two to three units should be cross-matched.
• *Antibiotics:* If there is known infection, or if a catheter has been in position, then antibiotics are always given to protect against septicaemia. It is still a matter of debate whether they are needed in every cold operation.

Postoperative care

• *The catheter:* After all forms of prostatectomy a catheter is left in the bladder, usually a three-way catheter which allows saline to run in and out of the bladder to dilute blood and prevent clots from blocking the catheter (Fig. 18.21). Some surgeons rely on natural formation of urine to irrigate the bladder, and encourage this with a diuretic. If a chip of prostate or a blood clot does block the catheter an attempt is made to wash it out with a bladder syringe using strict aseptic precautions. If this fails the catheter is removed and a new one is passed.

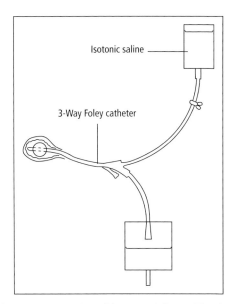

Isotonic saline

3-Way Foley catheter

Figure 18.21 Irrigation of the prostatic fossa with a three-way catheter.

• *Reactionary haemorrhage:* Reactionary haemorrhage may occur after any type of prostatectomy. The bladder fills with blood clot which cannot be evacuated with a bladder syringe. The patient is returned at once to the operating theatre where the clot is removed with an Ellik evacuator and the offending vessels are coagulated. Very occasionally the reactionary bleeding can be so furious that the only way to stop it is to open the retropubic space and pack the prostatic fossa.

• *Removal of the catheter:* All the bleeding has usually stopped within 24–48 hours, and the catheter is then removed. At first there may be some discomfort on passing urine, and an occasional leak if the patient coughs or strains. This soon recovers.

• *Going home:* Patients usually go home after 4 or 5 days, but the empty cavity from which the inner zone tissue has been removed is still raw and unhealed, and secondary haemorrhage may occur at any moment. It makes sense to advise him to avoid strain: a good rule is to do anything he ordinarily can do in his carpet slippers. Around the tenth postoperative day there is often a little haematuria. Patients understand this if it is explained beforehand that it may bleed a little when the 'scab' comes away. Very rarely the patient must be readmitted to have clot irrigated out of the bladder.

• *Recovery:* Recovery is not complete until the prostatic fossa has been completely relined with urothelium. This takes about 6 weeks. Until then the patient will notice some frequency and urgency, and the urine will continue to be a little cloudy, raising the suggestion of infection. Antibiotics are not needed, however, unless there is a significant growth of bacteria.

Chapter 19

Prostate cancer

Aetiology

There are unexplained differences in the incidence of prostate cancer in different parts of the world: it is relatively uncommon in men of Japanese and Indian ancestry, and more common in those of African ancestry. It is twice as common in men of African-American descent and is more likely to present at an advanced stage. The number of reported cases seems to be increasing, but this may be due to an increased awareness, the growing number of elderly men who are surviving, and better ways of making the diagnosis.

Incidence

Prostate cancer is the most common non-skin cancer in men. At the age of 50, about 15% of prostates contain islands of cancer; by the age of 80, the figure is nearly 100%. Prostate cancer accounts for less than 0.5% deaths in each age group over the age of 60. European age-standardised incidence and mortality for prostate cancer (EU estimates) are shown in Fig. 19.1. Introduction of the prostate-specific antigen (PSA) blood test in the late 1980s enhanced prostate cancer detection. A dramatic increase in the detection rate in the early 1990s was followed by a subsequent decline and

was thought to be due to detection of early small tumours. Cancer which is found by an elevated PSA or a prostate nodule on digital rectal examination is referred to as a clinical cancer. Cancer found only at autopsy is called a latent tumour. However, the total annual number of new cases shows an increase and this is frequently interpreted in an alarmist way to justify programmes of screening.

Pathology

Cancer usually arises in the peripheral zone which is usually compressed into a shell by benign enlargement of the central zone (Fig. 19.2). It is not uncommon that cancer does also arise in the inner zone.

Most prostate adenocarcinomas are composed of acini arranged in patterns variable in space, size and shape. Mucin and crytalloids are often present in the acinar lumens. The stroma frequently contains collagen. Perineural and microvascular invasion is a strong indicator of malignancy and correlates with histological grade.

Prostatic intraepithelial neoplasia

This pathological change is characterised by cellular proliferation within pre-existing ducts and acini with cytological changes mimicking cancer, including nuclear and nucleolar enlargement. Despite these changes, an intact or fragmented

Lecture Notes: Urology, 6th edition. By John Blandy and Amir Kaisary. Published 2009 by Blackwell Publishing. ISBN: 978-1-4051-2270-2.

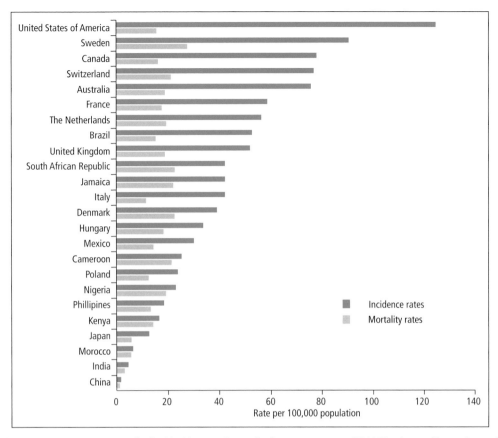

Figure 19.1 European age-standardised incidence and mortality for prostate cancer, EU 1998 estimates (Cancer Research in 2004).

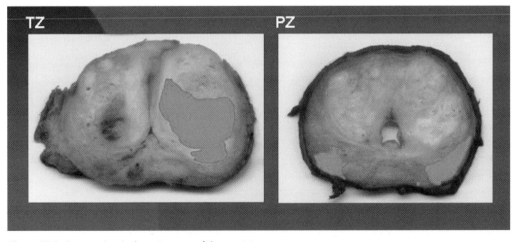

Figure 19.2 Cancer arises in the outer zone of the prostate.

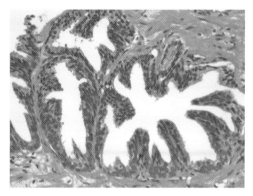

Figure 19.3 Prostaic intraepithelial neoplasia (PIN).

basal cell layer is retained unlike cancer where a basal cell layer is lacking. There are two grades: low-grade prostatic intraepithelial neoplasia (PIN) and high-grade PIN (Fig. 19.3). A high level of inter-observer variability with low-grade PIN limits its clinical value and indeed many pathologists do not report it. High-grade PIN is now generally accepted as a potential likely preinvasive stage of adenocarcinoma and its presence in prostate biopsies warrants repeat biopsy for concurrent or subsequent invasive adenocarcinoma.

Histological grade

The Gleason system is based on the assessment of the pattern of growth seen in two low-power fields (Figs. 19.4 and 19.5), each assigned a number from 1 to 5. The two numbers are added together to provide a Gleason sum score between 2 and 10. The Gleason system provides important prognostic information. It correlates very well with the clinical behaviour of the tumour and its response to treatment.

Tumour markers

Prostate-specific antigen

This is a protein secreted only by prostate cells whether benign or malignant. It is normally secreted into semen or lost in urine. It spills over into the bloodstream where it can be measured. It can also be detected by immunofluorescent methods in histological sections. Production of PSA by both normal and malignant prostate glands is dependent on male hormones (androgens) being present in the body at normal levels. The presence of an elevated PSA suggests that either the prostate is enlarged or an abnormal condition exists within it (inflammation, infection, trauma or cancer). An elevated PSA is not cancer specific.

Free and total PSA

PSA may exist in either a free form or one bound to proteins in the blood (alpha 2-macroglobulin or alpha 1-antichymotrypsin). For any given total PSA value with levels between 4 and 10 ng/mL, the chance of prostate cancer being present may be

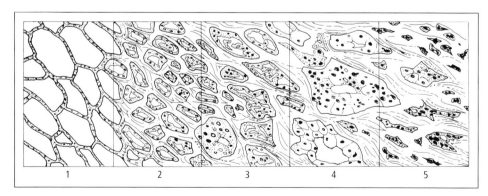

Figure 19.4 The Gleason system: for each tumour, two low-power fields are assigned a score from 1 to 5; the Gleason score is the sum.

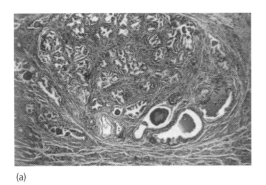
(a)

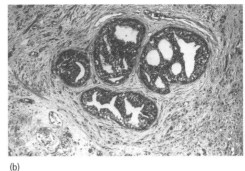
(b)

Figure 19.5 (a) Benign hyperplasia and (b) cancer – an area of Gleason 2 is surrounded by anaplastic Gleason 5.

Table 19.1 Total PSA age reference ranges.

Age range (years)	Reference range (ng/mL)
40–49	0–2.5
50–59	0–3.5
60–69	0–4.5
70–79	0–6.5

determined based on the percentage free PSA. For men with a percentage free PSA more than 25, the risk of prostate cancer being present may be so low that prostate biopsy may be avoided or delayed. This characteristic should not be used as a sole indicator and other factors such as the digital rectal examination should be taken into account.

Age-specific PSA levels

There is a consistent rise in the size of the prostate in the aging male (range 0.4–1.2 g/year). So, PSA increases with age (Table 19.1). The use of age-specific PSA levels enhances the specificity and sensitivity of the test and may avoid unnecessary biopsies. One should be suspicious of prostate cancer if the patient's age-specific PSA level is abnormal. The PSA cut-off levels are continuously being challenged in an attempt to improve prostate cancer detection at an earlier age and stage.

PSA density

An enlarged prostate gland of benign nature might produce an elevated PSA. In order to allow for the

contribution of benign hyperplasia, a calculation to enhance PSA specificity was proposed by dividing the serum PSA by prostate volume (cc). PSA density values more than 0.15, might indicate a risk of prostate cancer and prostate biopsy is recommended. There is no complete agreement in the literature about the accuracy of this tool, which many urologists consider useful.

PSA velocity

This is a measurement of change in PSA serum levels in nanograms per millilitre per year (ng/mL/year). A series of at least three PSA blood tests must be obtained. If the PSA increase is more than 0.75 ng/mL/year, one ought to suspect that prostate cancer might be causing the rise.

Doubling time

Evaluation of the rate of PSA change in men with prostate disease may provide a means to improve management. In patients with prostate cancer, PSA changes seem to have both a linear and an exponential phase. During the exponential phase, PSA doubling time for patients with local/regional carcinoma seem to range from 1.5 to 6.6 years (median 3 years). In those with advanced/metastatic disease, the range is 0.9 to 8.5 years (median 2 years). The PSA doubling time may be helpful in guiding the diagnosis and treatment of prostate cancer patients.

PCA3Plus

PCA3 gene is specific to the prostate cells and is over-expressed only by malignant tissue. It is significantly upregulated 60- to 100-fold in prostate cancer. Massaging the prostate gland releases prostate cells into the urinary tract where they can be collected in the first urine that is passed. The prostate cells are harvested and the expression of mRNA from the PCA3 gene assessed. PCA3 mRNA along with the mRNA of PSA is measured quantitatively and examined as a ratio. High ratios have been shown to be indicative of prostate cancer. It is of particular value in follow-up treatment of patients with an elevated serum PSA and negative biopsy results. The test has shown a sensitivity of 67% and a specificity of 89% claiming an overall accuracy of 81% for detection of prostate cancer in comparison to PSA of approximately 40%.

Staging of prostate cancer

Staging of prostate cancer takes into account its method of spread which is directly up into the bladder and seminal vesicles. It seldom goes through Denonvilliers' fascia into the rectum but instead can grow around it to cause obstruction. It quickly invades the pelvic lymph nodes, and spreads by veins and lymphatics into the marrow of the lumbar spine, pelvis and femora. The T staging in the TNM classification system is set out in Fig. 19.6.

Clinical presentation

Screening

Today carcinoma of the prostate is most often detected by screening with PSA. Knowing that little islands of cancer are present in most elderly men, it is surprising that cancer is not detected more often.

Chance finding at transurethral prostate resection

Carcinoma is found by chance in about 10% of patients undergoing transurethral resection of the prostate (TURP) for what was until then thought to be a benign enlargement of the prostate. Knowing the true incidence of cancer in the prostate, one would expect the figure to be higher, but of course TURP takes out mostly inner zone tissue, and spares the compressed outer zone where most of the cancers arise.

Local symptoms

• *Prostatism:* Compression of the urethra may cause symptoms identical with those due to benign enlargement.
• *Rectal obstruction:* If the cancer is encircling the rectum the patient may complain of pencil-thin stools and progressive constipation.
• *Uraemia:* Ureteric obstruction may lead to hydroureter and hydronephrosis and, if bilateral, to uraemia.

Distant metastases effects

Metastases may occur anywhere, but usually affect the lumbar vertebrae, pelvis and femora. These may cause bone pains, pathological fractures or spinal cord compression. In an X-ray these metastases are typically denser than the normal bone (osteosclerotic) because carcinoma of the prostate secretes *acid phosphatase*, an enzyme which lays down bone (Fig. 19.7). Osteolytic bone lesions are also found but much less often. Occasionally fibrinolysins produced by metastases can cause bruising and haemorrhages; anaemia is not uncommon.

Soft tissue metastases lead to symptoms according to the affected site, e.g. chronic cough in lung metastases disease.

Investigations

Transrectal ultrasound

The echogenicity of the prostate is determined by the amount of calcium in the tissues, which in

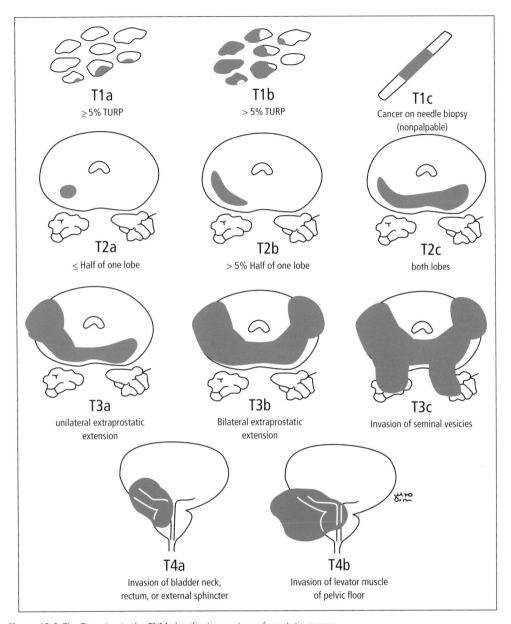

Figure 19.6 The T staging in the TNM classification system of prostatic cancer.

cancer may be greater or lesser than normal (Fig. 19.8). Any suspicious area is biopsied using a biopsy needle placed under ultrasonic control. Often a prostate harbouring cancerous changes shows normal echogenic features where the examination is driven by an elevated PSA value in the presence of a normal digital rectal examination.

Antibiotic prophylaxis therapy is routinely given and the complications of bleeding or infection are rare. Local anaesthesia may be given. The biopsies are obtained in a predetermined pattern to sample the peripheral zone. Transition zone biopsies are added when necessary. The ultrasound image may show that cancer has invaded the seminal

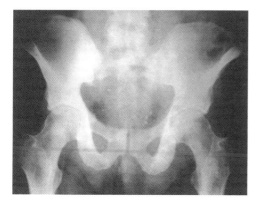

Figure 19.7 X-ray of pelvis showing areas of increased density caused by metastases.

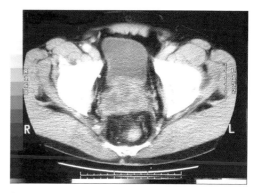

Figure 19.9 CT scan showing carcinoma of the prostate with impending ureteric obstruction due to extraprostatic invasion of the bladder base.

vesicles or the peri-prostatic fat and so help to stage the case. At the time of biopsy, determination of the prostate size and shape is obtained and any anatomical abnormalities are detected.

Computed tomography

The computed tomography (CT) scan may reveal enlarged pelvic lymph nodes and invasion of the seminal vesicles (Fig. 19.9) as well as spread of cancer to the liver and other organs.

Magnetic resonance imaging

This relies on the characteristics of tissues to provide two-dimensional pictures with different orientations. These images may be even more precise in staging the cancer and are often performed when radical prostatectomy is contemplated (Fig. 19.10).

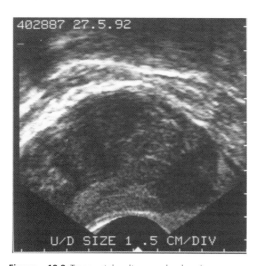

Figure 19.8 Transrectal ultrasound showing cancer breaching the capsule on the left side.

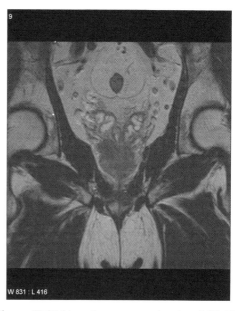

Figure 19.10 Magnetic resonance imaging (MRI) T2-weighted image showing invasion of the seminal vesicle on the right side.

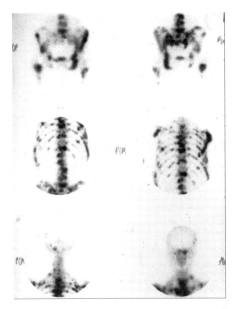

Figure 19.11 Bone scan showing multiple 'hot spots' from metastases.

Bone scan

The radionuclide ^{99m}Tc-MDP (methylene diphosphonate) is taken up by bone in proportion to the blood flow, so the increased vascularity of a metastasis shows a 'hot spot' (Fig. 19.11). False-positives are common from osteoarthritis and old fractures of the ribs. When the bones are so very widely invaded as to be almost uniform there may be a 'superscan'.

Treatment

Management of prostate cancer is dependent on the man who is diagnosed to have prostate cancer. Characters recognised include familial history, ethnic origin, life expectancy and the disease stage whether localised or metastatic. Involving the patient in view of the considerable debate that exists as to the preferred choice of treatment, the pros and cons of each different method of treatment should be explained so that an informed choice can be made. To advise patients one must be able to predict the outcome of each method of treatment. Here a nomogram may be helpful. A nomogram is a graphic representation of a statistical model that incorporates several variables to predict a particular end point. Predictive pre-treatment nomograms make outcome predictions based on the characteristics of individual patient: clinical stage, biopsy Gleason sum, pre-treatment PSA level, receipt of neoadjuvant hormonal deprivation therapy and total radiation dose as predictor variables. An example is shown in Table 19.2. Some men find it repugnant to think that they might be walking around with cancer. Others find the prospect of incontinence and impotence no less undesirable and prefer to take their chance.

Table 19.2 Prostate nomogram.

Prostate nomogram results – pre-treatment			
Pre-treatment PSA	9.1	Organ-confined disease	49%
Biopsy primary Gleason	3	Extra-capsular penetration	40%
Biopsy secondary Gleason	4	Seminal vesicle involvement	8%
Biopsy Gleason sum	7	Lymph node involvement	3%
1992 clinical tumour stage	T1C	5 years progression-free probability radical prostatectomy	77%
1997 clinical tumour stage	T1C		
Prescribed external radiation dose (64.8–86.4 Gy)	86.4	5 years progression-free probability external beam radical therapy	87%
Neoadjuvant hormones	No	5 years progression-free probability brachytherapy	72%
Neoadjuvant radiation	No		

High	Intermediate	Low
Clinical T3	Clinical T2 with	Clinical T2 with
Clinical T2 and PSA	PSA 10.1–20	PSA ≤ 10
>20	Or	And
Radiation failure pre-RT > T2b	Gleason score > 7	Gleason score ≥ 7
Gleason score ≤ 7		

Table 19.3 Predictive risk groups' criteria in prostate cancer.

Localised disease

Taking into account the prognostic parameters that have been identified, patients are divided into risk groups: high, intermediate and low (Table 19.3). The options in localised prostate cancer include watchful waiting/active surveillance, surgery, irradiation and methods of ablation including cryosurgery and high-intensity focused ultrasound.

Watchful waiting/active surveillance

In certain patients a policy of observation and monitoring might be a preferred management option. In an incidental prostate cancer found at transurethral prostate resection (T1a) the probability of disease progression may be very low. Patients who have reduced life expectancy might be monitored with regular PSA measurements, proceeding to therapy only if there was clear evidence of disease progression. Gleason histological grading is believed to be the best indicator of the probability of significant disease progression.

Radical prostatectomy

There is a heated debate between those who favour radical prostatectomy for cancers that appear to be confined to the prostate, and those who are against it.

The arguments in favour of radical surgery are:
• More of those who survive for 10–15 years after radical surgery do so without residual cancer.
• Radical prostatectomy avoids the misery of local recurrence in the pelvis.
• Improved surgical techniques can achieve potency preservation and continence.

The arguments against radical prostatectomy are:
• Almost every elderly man has a small cancer in his prostate, but less than 0.5% die of it; i.e., 99.5% do not.
• The only prospective controlled studies to have been carried out showed no differences in survival after 20 years between men treated by radical surgery or surveillance.
• Larger retrospective studies of Medicare patients show no difference in survival between those undergoing radical surgery and surveillance.
• The morbidity of radical prostatectomy includes incontinence, stricture and impotence in a (debated but large) proportion of patients.

Staging lymph node dissection

Most surgeons consider that radical prostatectomy is futile if the lymph nodes are involved and usually sample the lymph nodes around the obturator nerve and vessels before going ahead with radical surgery. This can be performed laparoscopically a few days before surgery is planned, or as the first stage of an open operation.

Radical prostatectomy

The prostate is approached through a lower abdominal incision. The lymph nodes along the internal iliac and obturator vessels are dissected and sent for frozen section, unless this has already been done. The dorsal veins of the penis are doubly ligated and divided behind the symphysis, and the neurovascular bundles going to the penis are pushed aside out of harm's way (Fig. 19.12). The urethra is transected, and the prostate lifted up, to reveal the seminal vesicles, whose vessels are

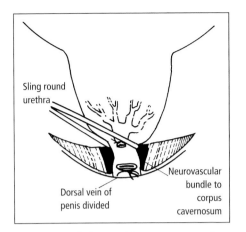

Figure 19.12 Radical retropubic prostatectomy: the neurovascular bundles to the penis can be preserved.

ligated. The bladder is then cut across at the level of the bladder neck, which is then narrowed, and sutured to the stump of the urethra over a catheter (Fig. 19.13).

Transperineal prostatectomy is a different surgical approach offered to selected patients where no lymphadenectomy is contemplated. Laparoscopic radical prostatectomy is an approach gaining wide appeal. Both techniques rely on the expertise of the urological surgeon and meticulous patient selection.

Open retropubic surgical excision is gradually now being challenged by laparoscopic and robotic techniques.

Radiotherapy

There are numerous ways to deliver therapeutic radiation including external beam radiotherapy with the linear accelerator and brachytherapy (inserting radioactive sources into the prostate under transrectal ultrasound control (Fig. 19.14). There is no clear consensus as to which method of radiotherapy is best. What is clear is that certain patients may be better suited for one or another or, in fact, a combination of these modalities. Pretreatment PSA levels and Gleason histological score are very important tools for prediction of response. It is important to define the patient's risk status (high, intermediate or low) to determine the method of choice offered to the individual patient. No randomised prospective controlled study has ever shown that any type of radiation is better or worse than surveillance or radical prostatectomy. Survival is much the same, but residual cancer is found more often after radiation in the survivors than in those treated by surgery, even though it does not necessarily cause symptoms. Neoadjuvant and adjuvant hormone suppression combined with radiotherapy improves local control, may prolong disease-free survival, and may delay the time to the development of metastatic disease and extend overall survival in some subsets of patients.

Painful proctitis is a common early sequel of radiation, and impotence occurs in a proportion, probably as a result of radiation arteritis.

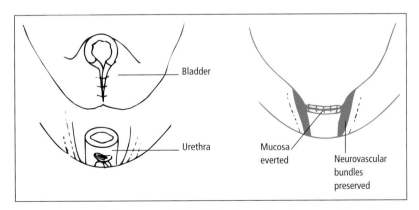

Figure 19.13 After the prostate has been removed, the bladder is sutured to the stump of the urethra.

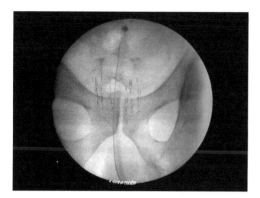

Figure 19.14 Brachytherapy.

Cryosurgery

Complete cell destruction occurs in response to freezing down to temperatures reaching $-40°C$. The direct effects of cryosurgery on cells include:
• Crystallisation of extracellular fluid leading to cellular dehydration.
• Cellular pH changes leading to electrolyte abnormalities resulting in denaturation of cellular proteins.
• Lipoproteins are damaged in response to the thermal shock.
• Cellular membrane disruption occurs as a result of intracellular crystallisation.
• Membrane disruption occurs due to fluid influx during thawing following freezing.
• Thrombosis and vascular stasis occurs after freezing.

Cryosurgery clinical experience continues to advance. Improvements and refinement of the delivery systems are promising and may lead to increase in its use.

High-intensity focused ultrasound therapy

A recent method of treatment carried out under a spinal or general anaesthetic is thought to be offering an advance in prostate cancer management. A beam of ultrasound emission from a rectal probe targets the prostate gland. It is focused to reach a high intensity in the target tissue where absorption of the ultrasound energy creates an increase in the temperature which destroys tissue. A cooling balloon surrounds the probe to protect the rectal mucosa from the high temperature. A urethral or a suprapubic catheter is inserted after the procedure to aid urinary drainage during the time the necrotic debris is expelled. The long-term clinical outcome, safety and efficacy, reduction in PSA levels, post-treatment biopsy findings, survival and impact on quality of life are being audited.

Advanced/metastatic disease
Hormonal manipulation

Malignant prostate cells start off by requiring a daily supply of testosterone without which they die. In cancer, mutant clones eventually emerge which no longer depend on testosterone, and this (on average) occurs in about 80% of men within 2 years of the diagnosis of metastases; however, among the 20% who do not develop metastases within 2 years there are many who survive for decades without any other treatment. Largely as a result of these and other anecdotal experiences, there was a feeling that no harm arose from deferring the treatment until metastases began to cause symptoms. This was the subject of a recent Medical Research Council controlled prospective trial but this showed an unacceptably high incidence of serious metastatic complications in patients for whom hormone therapy had been deferred.

The different ways of hormonal manipulation and the adverse effects encountered are illustrated in Fig. 19.15. The testosterone metabolic pathway in Fig. 19.16 demonstrates the effects of withdrawal of testosterone and its metabolites or antagonism for the metabolites only on target tissue. The supply of testosterone can be cut off or interfered within a number of ways:
• *Orchidectomy:* The testicles may be removed, or a subcapsular orchidectomy may be performed which leaves something behind which feels like a normal testicle.
• *Diethylstilboestrol:* This is a synthetic oestrogen which blocks the products of metabolism of testosterone. Given in large doses of 5 mg/day it had a high incidence of cardiovascular side effects but a dose of 1 mg daily seems to be just as effective without cardiovascular sequelae.

- *Luteinizing hormone-releasing hormone agonist:* Luteinizing hormone-releasing hormone (LHRH) overstimulates the anterior pituitary gland and initially more Luteinizing hormone is released during the first 2 weeks of treatment and thus an increased testosterone secretion. This may cause a 'flare-up' with pain and other complications from metastases; thus, LHRH agonists are given in combination with drugs which block the action of testosterone in the cells – anti-androgens (see below). However, downregulation of the prostate cell receptors leads to a decreased Luteinizing hormone production, which in turn results in the testis no longer secreting testosterone with maintenance therapy.
- *Gonadotrophin-releasing hormone antagonist:* Recent interest in novel gonadotrophin-releasing hormone antagonist formulation is appealing as it can avoid the initial testosterone rise seen in the usage of LHRH agonist.
- *5-Alpha-reductase inhibitors:* 5-Alpha-reductase inhibitors, such as finasteride, prevent the activation of testosterone to dihydrotestosterone but they are seldom used in the treatment of prostate cancer.
- *Anti-androgens:* Dihydrotestosterone acts on receptors in the cytosol of the prostate cell. These receptors are blocked by two types of anti-androgen:
  - steroids such as megestrol and cyproterone; and
  - non-steroids such as flutamide, nilutamide and bicalutamide.

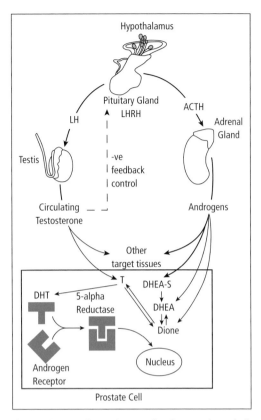

Figure 19.15 Androgen hormonal pathway and metabolic changes demonstrating sites of various treatment approaches.

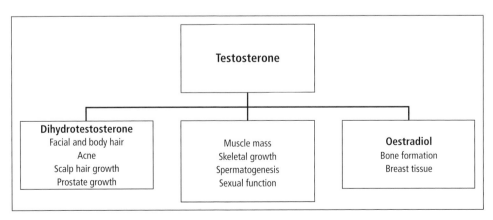

Figure 19.16 The testosterone metabolic pathway.

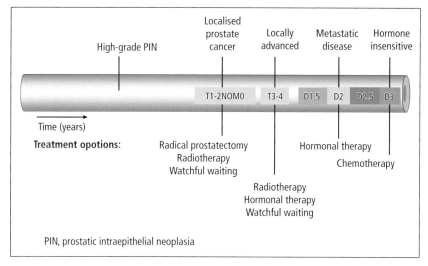

Figure 19.17 Prostate continuum.

• *Aromatase inhibitors:* These prevent the action of *aromatase*, an enzyme in the prostate cell which converts adrenal steroids into testosterone. They are still under trial.

Maximal androgen blockade

A combination of LHRH agonists given together with anti-androgens is claimed to give a small improvement (a matter of weeks) in survival but not everyone is convinced that this is justified by the side effects, let alone the expense of this additional therapy.

Radiotherapy

Isolated painful metastases respond dramatically to small doses of radiation, which can particularly be useful when there is a pathological fracture or spinal cord compression. Severe pain in the skeleton can be helped by hemi-body radiation, a technique in which one half of the body is irradiated, to control bony metastases. This also destroys the bone marrow in the irradiated bones, but after a few weeks to allow this marrow to be repopulated

by haematogenous cells from the rest of the bone, the other half is irradiated.

Similar relief of pain can be produced by radioactive phosphorus-32, strontium-89 and diphosphonate.

Chemotherapy

The development of hormone independence is observed in a majority of the patients at some time following androgen deprivation. Chemotherapy has been found to have limited relative value and a potential for toxicity, although some new drugs e.g. Docetaxel (Taxotere), show a satisfactory role in management of metastatic hormone-refractory prostate cancer with generally manageable and predictable adverse effects.

New approaches

Attempts at developing new treatment compounds are currently based on increased understanding of prostate cancer biology. Anti-sense compounds, tumour vaccines, endothelin antagonists and gene therapy are some of the current extensive clinical ongoing advances (see Fig. 19.17).

Chapter 20

The urethra

Anatomy

In both sexes the urethra is lined with urothelium near the bladder and squamous epithelium near the external meatus. In between is modified columnar epithelium. *Para-urethral glands* enter all along the urethra, secreting mucus. Some of these glands are of special importance.

In males the most important para-urethral glands make up the *prostate*: in addition there is a pair of *Cowper's* glands in the levator ani, and a pair of *Littré's* glands near the external meatus. Any of these may become infected and form an abscess (Fig. 20.1).

The urethra is surrounded by the corpus spongiosum which in males expands to form the glans penis. Each corpus spongiosum is supported by a pair of corpora cavernosa, which is attached to the medial aspect of the ischiopubic rami (Fig. 20.2).

In females the urethra is shorter, and surrounded by a sleeve of erectile corpus spongiosum which

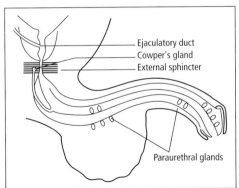

Figure 20.1 Anatomy of the male urethra.

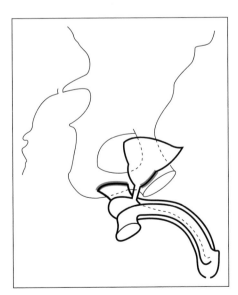

Figure 20.2 The fixed attachments of the corpora cavernosa to the ischiopubic rami below and the prostate to the symphysis pubis above: the membranous urethra is the weak link.

Lecture Notes: Urology, 6th edition. By John Blandy and Amir Kaisary. Published 2009 by Blackwell Publishing. ISBN: 978-1-4051-2270-2.

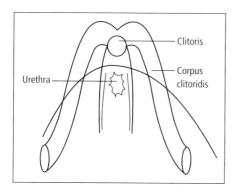

Figure 20.3 Anatomy of the female urethra and clitoris.

continues into the glans of the clitoris, flanked by two smaller corpora cavernosa (Fig. 20.3).

Sphincters

In males the three components of the sphincter surround the urethra at the bladder neck, the supramembranous sphincter and the levator ani.

In females there are the same three elements to the sphincter: the bladder neck, the intramural sleeve, made up of a mixture of striated and smooth muscle, and below this the levator ani (Fig. 20.4).

Congenital disorders of the urethr

Errors in the genital folds

Hypospadias

As the embryonic *genital folds* roll in to form the male urethra and corpus spongiosum, they may fail to fuse together, resulting in a urethra which opens on the underside of the penis – hypospadias. There are different degrees of hypospadias according to how far down the urethra the defect extends (Fig. 20.5).

Glandular hypospadias (Fig. 20.6): Here the urethra opens on the underside of the glans, but there is no other deformity. It causes no trouble in later life, and it is very questionable whether anything needs to be done about it at all. It can be corrected by an operation, but it is doubtful whether this is justified merely on the basis of some fancied cosmetic advantage.

Penile hypospadias: Here the urethra opens about half-way along the penis. Correction is necessary, and the important thing is to refer the baby to a paediatric urological centre where these operations are done often enough to give the team experience. As so often in paediatric urology, this is not a job for the occasional amateur who would like to have a try. In specialised centres a one-stage operation is often successful (Fig. 20.7).

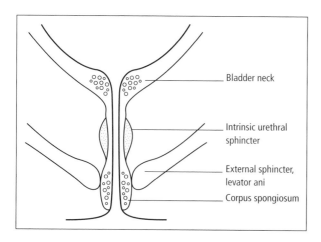

- Bladder neck
- Intrinsic urethral sphincter
- External sphincter, levator ani
- Corpus spongiosum

Figure 20.4 Structure of the female urethra.

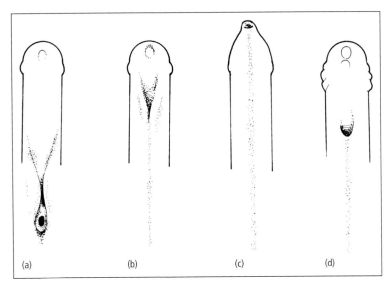

Figure 20.5 Incomplete inrolling of the genital folds results in different degrees of hypospadias.

Complete hypospadias: Correction of this deformity is even more difficult and referral to an expert, who can sometimes correct the deformity in one stage, is even more necessary.

Duplex urethra

Wrinkling of the genital folds as they roll in may give rise to a double urethra which is seldom complete. Sometimes the two channels communicate with the result that the lower one balloons out and obstructs urination – the so-called *anterior urethral valve* (Fig. 20.8).

Errors in the development of the cloacal membrane

These are dealt with under exstrophy and epispadias.

Congenital posterior urethral valves

The embryological explanation of this anomaly remains a mystery. There is a thin tough membrane

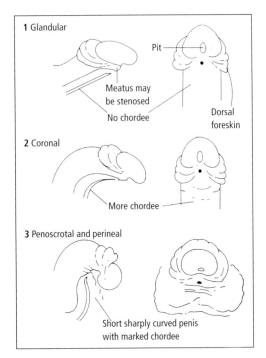

Figure 20.6 Varying degrees of hypospadias.

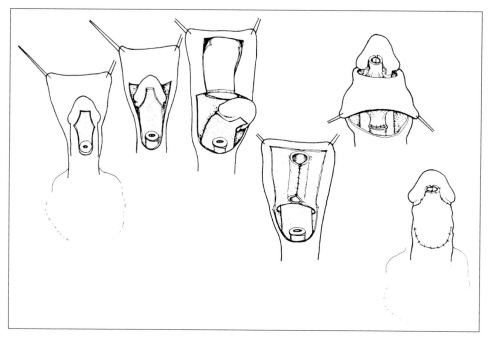

Figure 20.7 One-stage operation for hypospadias.

just below the verumontanum, with a hole in it like a parachute (Fig. 20.9). It causes obstruction. The bladder goes through all the phases of obstruction responding with hypertrophy, trabeculation and so on, followed by failure. If the condition is detected in the foetus by ultrasound scanning, a grommet may be inserted between the distended bladder and the amniotic cavity to relieve the pressure.

Prune-belly syndrome

The distended bladder of the foetus squeezes the abdominal wall and prevents ingrowth of muscle from either side so that the belly is thin and wrinkled. The testicles cannot descend. By the time the baby boy is born the valve may be intact, but sometimes it has ruptured, leaving the prune-belly without an explanation (Fig. 20.10). Spontaneous cure has been recorded in utero when serial ultrasound scans suddenly show the huge bladder to have disappeared.

Treatment. Once the child has been delivered, nothing is easier than to destroy the little membrane with a hook equipped with diathermy (Fig. 20.11).

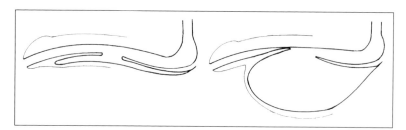

Figure 20.8 Duplication of the urethra – anterior urethral valve.

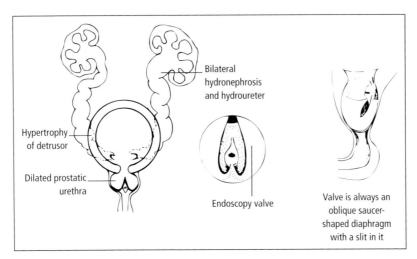

Bilateral
hydronephrosis
and hydroureter

Hypertrophy
of detrusor

Dilated prostatic
urethra

Endoscopy valve

Valve is always an
oblique saucer-
shaped diaphragm
with a slit in it

Figure 20.9 Congenital posterior urethral valves.

Trauma

Iatrogenic trauma

Instrumental injury to the urethra is very common. A clean cut will heal with an inconspicuous scar, and no stricture. When the injury is caused by pressure of a catheter leading to ischaemic necrosis – essentially a bedsore – healing leads to a stricture. These are typically found near the meatus, at the penoscrotal junction, or at the external sphincter (Fig. 20.12).

There is one important variation on this theme. After open heart or aortic surgery multiple strictures may occur along the length of the urethra. At first these were thought to be caused by some toxic chemical in latex catheters. Later the same kind of stricture, though less common, was seen with other types of catheter. It is now thought that the strictures are due to a combination of ischaemia (while the circulation is suspended) and pressure of the catheter, perhaps made worse by chemicals in the material of the catheter itself (Fig. 20.13).

Perineal injury

In past times many a jack tar would fall from the rigging of a sailing ship astride a spar, or a Johnny Head-in-Air would trip over a man-hole cover in the street. Today the injury occurs in sport and industry. The blunt force compresses the bulbar urethra up against the inferior edge of the symphysis and tears the corpus spongiosum and urethra (Fig. 20.14). Because the corpus spongiosum is firmly attached to the corpora cavernosa its ends do not retract (Fig. 20.15). Urine and blood escape into the scrotum, in a space which is limited by the fasciae of Scarpa and Colles. The concentrated or infected urine may cause necrosis of the fat and overlying skin (Fig. 20.16). In neglected cases the entire skin of the scrotum and penis may slough away, leaving only the testes preserved by the blood supply of the spermatic cord.

Management

The first priority is to prevent urine escaping into the scrotum. A suprapubic tube is put in the bladder as an emergency. If there is a collection of urine and blood in the scrotum it must be drained, but no attempt is made to repair the urethra at this stage.

About 10 days later the urethra is examined with the flexible cystoscope: in nearly every case it will

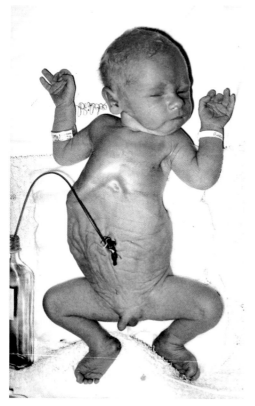

Figure 20.10 Prune-belly syndrome. (Courtesy of the late Mr J.H. Johnston.)

be found to have healed completely. Occasionally the scar shrinks and causes a stricture, but it is always short and easy to treat.

Fractured pelvis with rupture of the membranous urethra

The membranous urethra is very thin and connects two fixed points, the prostate above, which is firmly attached to the symphysis, and the bulbar urethra below, which is bound to the corpora cavernosa on either side: these are in turn fixed to the ischiopubic ramus. If a fracture separates these two fixed points the membranous urethra is first stretched, and may be torn across completely. There are three types of injury: (i) minimal displacement of the pelvis; (ii) gross displacement of the pelvis; and (iii) combined urethral and rectal injuries.

Minimal displacement of the pelvis

When the pelvic ring is compressed from front to back, e.g. by a car backing into a man leaning over a wall, it gives way where it is thinnest – at the pubic and ischial rami on either side of the symphysis (Fig. 20.17). The symphysis carries the prostate back with it while the bulbar urethra remains attached to the ischiopubic rami. The membranous urethra is first stretched, and may be torn completely or incompletely. The car backs off and the pelvic ring springs back almost to its original position, but in practice the symphysis ends up being displaced a little posteriorly to its original position. If the lumen of the urethra is intact it will

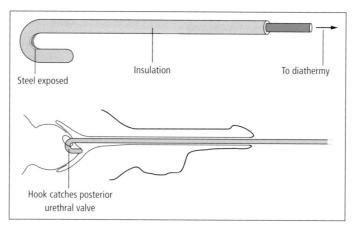

Steel exposed   Insulation   To diathermy

Hook catches posterior urethral valve

Figure 20.11 Insulated diathermy hook for destroying posterior urethral valve.

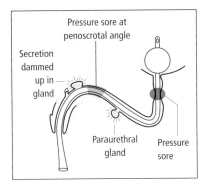

Figure 20.12 Dangers of a snugly fitting catheter.

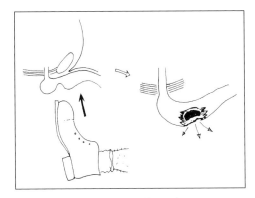

Figure 20.14 Perineal injury to the urethra.

now have an S-shaped bend. If torn completely, the prostatic urethra will come to lie behind the bulb (Fig. 20.18).

Management

In the accident and emergency department X-rays show the typical fracture. Blood escaping from the urethra shows that there has been some damage. Using sterile precautions, about 20 mL of soluble contrast medium is gently injected into the ure-

thra: extravasation confirms that the urethra has been damaged. *At this stage, do not try to pass a catheter: put in a suprapubic tube.*

The next step depends on the general state of the patient. Usually there are other more important injuries to be taken care of and it takes several days for the patient to recover sufficiently for the urethral injury to be investigated. A flexible cystoscope is passed. In an *incomplete injury* the way can be seen into the bladder and nothing more

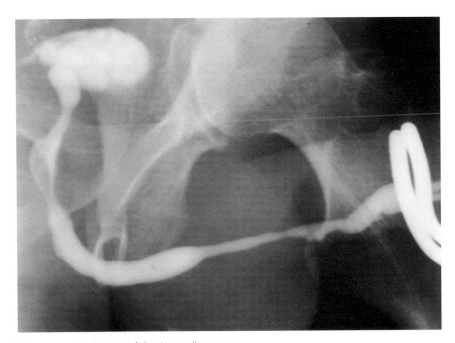

Figure 20.13 Long urethral stricture following cardiac surgery.

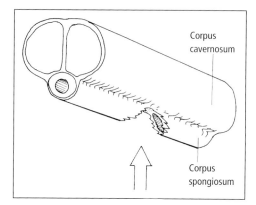

Figure 20.15 The attachments to the corpora cavernosa prevent the ends of the injured urethra from retracting.

need be done at this stage. About 2 weeks later the cystoscopy is repeated and at worst may show the S-shaped bend whose thin septa can easily be incised (Fig. 20.19).

If the urethra has been *completely* torn and the flexible cystoscope does not show any way into the bladder, the bulbar urethra is exposed through a perineal incision, the haematoma is evacuated, and the separated ends are anastomosed together over a silicone catheter (Fig. 20.20). The sooner this can be done the easier it is, but the timing of this operation is nearly always determined by the patient's other injuries.

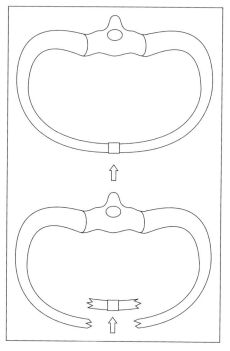

Figure 20.17 Anteroposterior injury: the pelvic ring gives way at its thinnest part.

Gross displacement of the pelvis

Here the anatomy of the injury is different. The patient has usually been driving a car with an outstretched lower limb, and the force of the impact

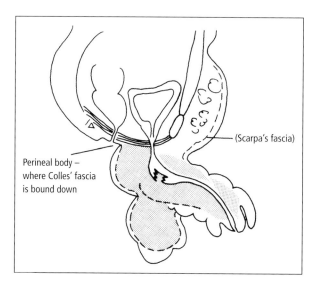

Figure 20.16 Urine and blood escape into the scrotum and perineum.

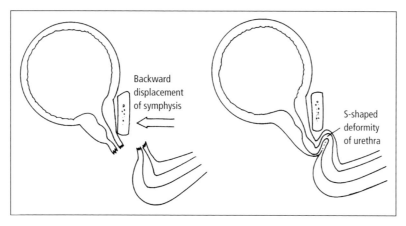

Figure 20.18 The displaced segment of pelvic ring returns almost to its original position but the prostatic end now lies posterior to the bulbar end of the ruptured urethra.

is transmitted along the limb, forcing the head of the femur through the acetabulum, and dislocating one half of the pelvis upwards, fracturing the pubic and ischial rami and dislocating the sacroiliac joint (Fig. 20.21). The half pelvis carries up the bladder and prostate. If the bulbar urethra rides up as well, then the urethra may escape damage, but more often the bulbar urethra remains attached to the opposite half of the pelvis and the membranous urethra is torn across. The gap between the severed ends of the urethra is now equal to the distance between the dislocated halves of the pelvis.

Management

In this type of injury the two halves of the pelvis do not spring back together: on the contrary, reduc-tion can be very difficult. There is always severe internal haemorrhage from torn pelvic vessels as well as other major injuries, e.g. to the head, liver and chest. For the first 48 hours the priority is *re-suscitation* and saving life. One of the best ways to limit the internal bleeding is to reduce the dislocated pelvis, and maintain the correct position with an external fixator (Fig. 20.22).

A urethrogram performed (as above) in the accident and emergency department will show whether or not the urethra is damaged. If there is no extravasation, it is safe to pass a urethral catheter. But if there is extravasation, or if there is any doubt, it is better to put in a suprapubic tube. This can be difficult in the presence of the pelvic haematoma, but is greatly helped by using

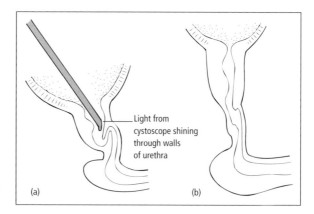

Figure 20.19 Urethroscopy may show an S-shaped bend, whose walls can be incised.

(a)   (b)

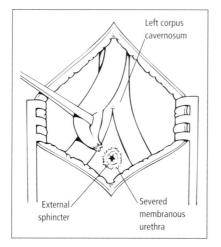

Figure 20.20 End-to-end anastomosis of the ruptured urethra through a perineal approach.

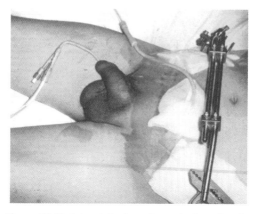

Figure 20.22 External fixation after reduction of a displaced fracture of the pelvis.

ultrasound to locate the bladder and make sure the suprapubic tube is in the right position.

Correct reduction of the dislocated pelvis will bring the separated ends of the urethra nearly together. When the general condition of the patient permits, a combination of cystogram and urethrogram (an 'up-and-down-a-gram') shows where the separated ends of the urethra are lying and an op-

eration is performed to anastomose them together. The timing of this operation is determined by the general condition of the patient, and it is seldom possible for several weeks.

The bulbar urethra is mobilised through a perineal incision, and the prostatic urethra exposed through a retropubic incision. In practice the prostate may have to be mobilised so that the torn ends can be brought together without tension (Fig. 20.23).

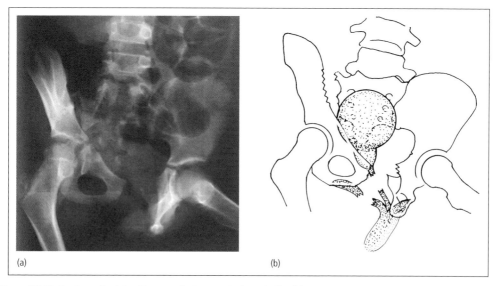

(a)   (b)

Figure 20.21 Fracture of pelvis with gross displacement of one half-pelvis.

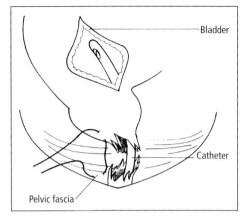

Figure 20.23 It may be necessary to mobilise the prostate through a retropubic approach.

Unreduced dislocation

Sometimes it proves to be impossible to effect an accurate reduction of the dislocated half pelvis, and by the time the patient is ready to undergo any urological reconstruction, the pelvis is fixed and the severed ends of the urethra are separated by a long gap. To reconstruct this is exceedingly difficult. Essentially part of the malunited callus has to be removed to allow the mobilised bulbar urethra to be brought up to the lower end of the prostate. There are a number of different methods for doing this, which indicates that none of them is always successful (Fig. 20.24).

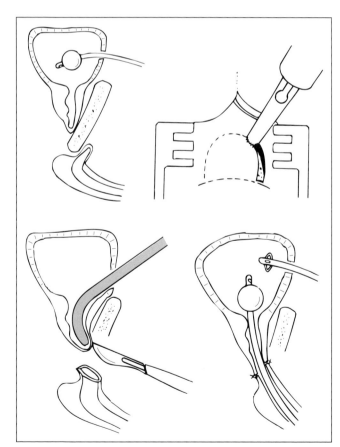

Figure 20.24 Unreduced displaced fracture of pelvis: end-to-end anastomosis after removing a window of symphysis.

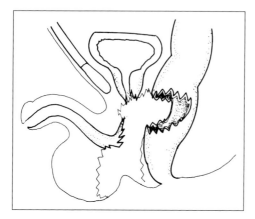

Figure 20.25 Massive crush injury with laceration of rectum.

Combined urethral and rectal injuries

Combined urethral and rectal injuries may be caused by gun-shot wounds which are rare and very dangerous. In civilian cases the cause is usually a rolling-crushing injury (Fig. 20.25). If the rectum is torn, it is essential that faeces are diverted as soon as possible or clostridial infection is likely to lead to gas gangrene. A colostomy is performed and the distal colon and rectum thoroughly washed out. A careful débridement of the wound is performed, bleeding controlled, and a suprapubic tube inserted. The wound is packed. *No attempt is made to perform a primary suture.* Plans can then be made for secondary suture and delayed reconstruction.

Complications of urethral injuries

Stricture: Stricture is a common result of any type of urethral injury.

Impotence: Impotence can occur after pelvic fractures without urethral injury, and is caused by damage to the neurovascular bundle of the penis or the pelvic autonomic nerves by the fracture and dislocation of the pelvic bones.

Impaired ejaculation: Damage to the sympathetic nerves may cause paralysis of the bladder neck and seminal vesicles resulting in retrograde or dry ejaculation.

Incontinence: If the bladder neck has been denervated or destroyed, or if the supramembranous intramural sphincter is damaged by the injury, then the patient may be incontinent.

Inflammation of the urethra

Gonorrhoea has been with mankind from time immemorial. Pharaohs took catheters with them to the after-life, and Socrates made jokes about it. Infection with *Neisseria gonorrhoeae* causes acute inflammation in the periurethral glands. There is a profuse discharge of yellow pus in which a Gram stain will show the typical Gram-negative intracellular diplococci. The patient suffers painful urination, and the oedema and inflammation may cause the penis to bend when erect – *chaudepisse cordée*. Eventually the inflammation subsides, but if not treated promptly with antibiotics, leads to scarring in the periurethral tissues which contracts and causes a stricture (Fig. 20.26). There are other bacterial causes of urethritis, notably *Chlamydia trachomatis*, in which the organism is more difficult to identify, but which can also progress to a stricture.

Clinical features of a stricture

The symptoms of a urethral stricture are those of outflow obstruction, indistinguishable from those caused by an enlarged prostate.

Physical signs

There are usually no physical signs, but in long-standing strictures palpation of the urethra will reveal thickening and induration in the corpus spongiosum.

Complications of a stricture

Urinary infection: Infected urine upstream of the stricture, whatever the cause, may be forced into the paraurethral ducts proximal to the stricture and cause further urethritis, with a progression of the stricture along the urethra (Fig. 20.27).

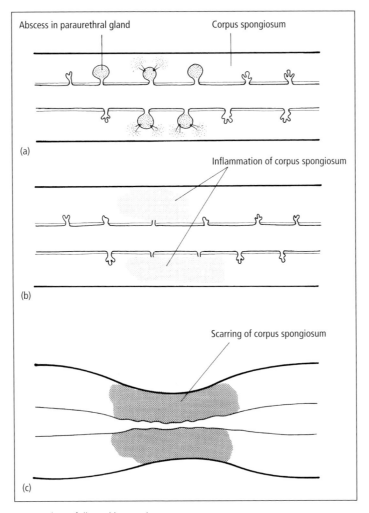

Figure 20.26 Acute gonorrhoea followed by scarring.

Para-urethral abscess: An infected para-urethral gland may suppurate, and pus may point in the scrotum, and after it has been incised or has discharged, urine may leak through a fistula. When these are multiple the result is a 'watering-can perineum'. Stones may form in these fistulae (Fig. 20.28).

Sterility: Even though urine may flow, the thicker semen may be obstructed by the stricture and lead to sterility.

Cancer: In strictures that have been present for many years, especially when complicated by fistulae, squamous cell cancer may arise.

Investigations

A flow rate will document the progress of a stricture, but may give a false reassurance that all is well since flow is proportional to the square of the diameter of the urethra.

Urethrography using a water-soluble contrast medium shows the stricture (Fig. 20.29), the fibrous changes in the corpus spongiosum, are better imaged with ultrasound scan (Fig. 20.30).

The flexible cystoscope is an easy way to examine the stricture directly.

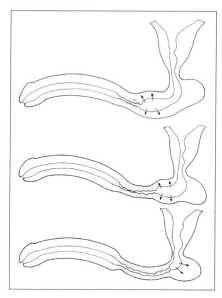

Figure 20.27 Progression of a stricture.

Treatment

Regular intermittent dilatation: This is the traditional method of managing a stricture. Ancient instruments were adapted from wax tapers, and the best wax came from the Algerian port of Bujiyah, so flexible dilators are still called *bougies* even though they are nowadays made of plastic not wax. Curved polished steel dilators are usually called *sounds* because they resemble the ancient instrument used before the days of X-rays, to 'sound' for stone in the bladder (Fig. 20.31). Whether flexible or rigid, dilators come in sets of gradually increasing size. They are used to stretch the stricture. Today, patients are given a self-lubricating catheter which they pass on themselves to keep the stricture dilated just as they used to do in ancient Greece.

Internal urethrotomy: When a stricture is too tight to allow a dilator to be passed, the scar tissue is incised under vision with the Sachse optical urethrotome (Fig. 20.32). Urethrotomy is then followed up by regular self-catheterisation.

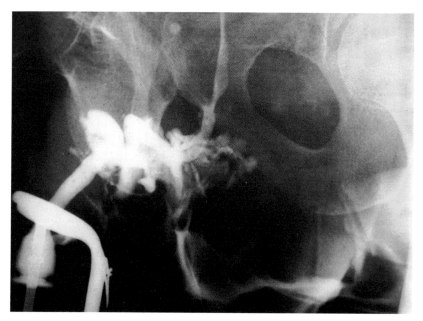

Figure 20.28 Multiple fistulae after a stricture – watering-can perineum.

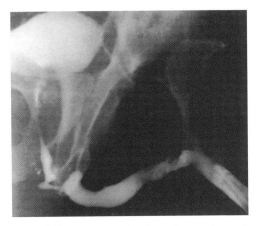

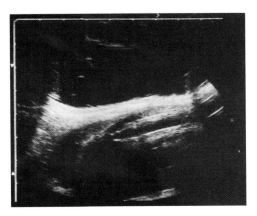

Figure 20.29 Urethrogram showing typical post-traumatic stricture with backward displacement of upper prostatic part.

Figure 20.30 Ultrasound image of urethra showing peri-urethral fibrosis. (Courtesy of Dr W. Hately.)

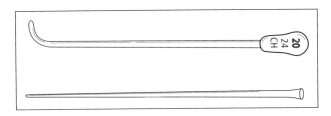

Figure 20.31 Urethral sound and bougie.

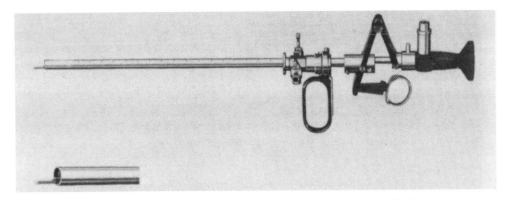

Figure 20.32 Sachse optical urethrotome. (Courtesy of Messrs Rimmer Bros, UK Agents for Karl Storz.)

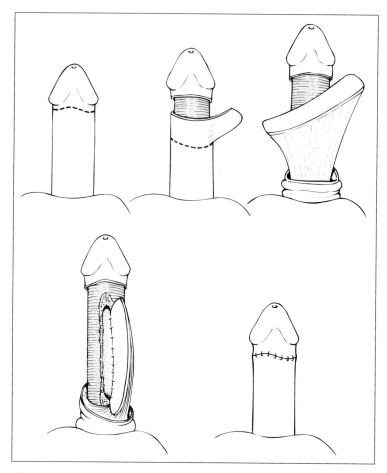

Figure 20.33 Pedicled skin graft urethroplasty.

Urethroplasty: To prevent scar tissue from contracting after burns in the skin, plastic surgeons apply a skin graft, and there are many ways of adapting this principle to the urethra. The graft can be made of buccal mucosa, split skin or whole thickness skin used as a free graft or on a pedicle of dartos (Fig. 20.33). There are many variations of this principle and the fact that there are so many is sufficient evidence that none of them is completely successful. Urethroplasty is only used when urethrotomy and regular dilatation fail to keep the stricture well controlled.

Chapter 21

The penis

Surgical anatomy

The penis is made of the two corpora cavernosa and the corpus spongiosum surrounding the urethra which expands to form the glans penis (Fig. 21.1). All three are surrounded by the tough rubbery Buck's fascia. When they fill with blood there is an erection. The spongy spaces of the corpora are made of compartments lined with smooth muscle: those of the two corpora cavernosa intercommunicate freely, but not with the corpus spongiosum and glans.

The glans penis is developed from the genital tubercle, into which a tunnel is formed during the last stage of the embryological development of the penis. Sometimes this tunnel is imperfect, leading to glandular hypospadias.

A hood of skin then grows over the glans to form the prepuce, and in the later months of foetal life, this hood becomes adherent to the glans. This congenital adherence breaks down spontaneously during the first few years of childhood and almost never causes any trouble.

Circumcision

The ancient religious rite of circumcision is of great anthropological interest, but is not indicated

Lecture Notes: Urology, 6th edition. By John Blandy and Amir Kaisary. Published 2009 by Blackwell Publishing. ISBN: 978-1-4051-2270-2.

on any surgical grounds and is followed by many complications. The arguments for and against neonatal circumcision have been raging for many centuries, with passion inversely proportional to evidence.

True phimosis, i.e. where there is obstruction to the escape of urine from the preputial space, is very rare, and easily dealt with by a small incision in the narrow meatus – preputioplasty (Fig. 21.2).

Balanitis, recurrent inflammation behind a prepuce that cannot be retracted after the age of 5 or 6, can be dealt with by circumcision or preputioplasty, but can usually be avoided by gentle retraction of the prepuce in the bath.

Blood supply

Arteries

The penis receives blood from three terminal branches of the internal pudendal artery (Fig. 21.3) on each side: the deep arteries of the corpora, the dorsal arteries and the bulbourethral arteries.

Veins

There are three groups of veins (Fig. 21.4):
• The *deep dorsal* veins drain the corpora cavernosa and lead under the symphysis pubis into the large veins which surround the prostate and bladder.

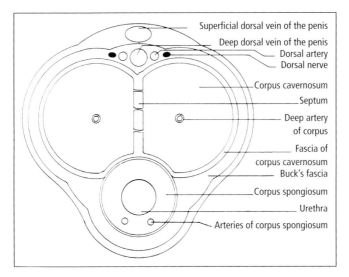

Figure 21.1 Transverse section through the penis.

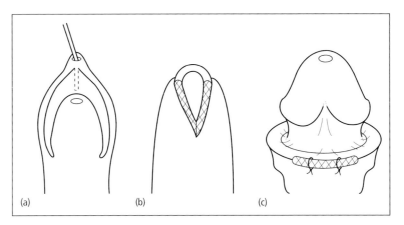

Figure 21.2 Preputioplasty.

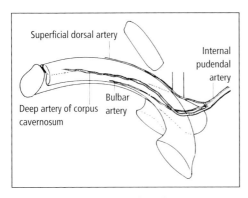

Figure 21.3 Arterial blood supply to the penis.

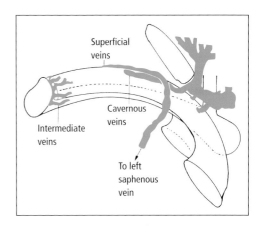

Figure 21.4 Venous drainage of the penis.

- The *superficial* veins, under the skin, mostly drain into the saphenous veins.
- The *intermediate* veins, deep to Buck's fascia, drain blood from the glans penis into both deep and superficial systems.

Nerves

Sensation

Sensation from the penis is carried in the dorsal nerves which run beside each dorsal artery to join the pudendal nerve (S2, S3).

Motor nerves

The cavernous nerves carry *parasympathetic* fibres in two discrete bundles on either side of the prostate, surrounding the arteries. Care is taken to preserve them in the operation of radical nerve-sparing prostatectomy.

Physiology of erection

There are three phases:
- *Flaccid state:* The flaccid penis has a relatively low blood flow through its spongy tissues.
- *Tumescence:* Parasympathetic stimulation, mediated by neurotransmitter substances (whose action is imitated by papaverine, phentolamine and prostaglandin E), causes the small branches of the deep arteries of the corpora cavernosa to dilate and fill the spaces of the spongy tissue with blood, while their smooth muscle walls relax. This relaxation is effected by *cyclic guanosine monophosphate*, which in turn is degraded by *phosphodiesterase*. The pressure inside the corpus cavernosum rises to about 40 mm Hg (Fig. 21.5).
- *Rigidity:* During the third phase of erection further parasympathetic stimulation occludes the veins leading out of the corpora cavernosa and spongiosum trapping blood inside them. The pressure rises inside the corpora to over 150 mm Hg.

Ejaculation

There are five steps in ejaculation (Fig. 21.6). The first four are under autonomic control: the fifth is mediated by somatic motor components in the pudendal nerve:
- the seminal vesicles pump themselves up;
- the bladder neck contracts;
- the vas deferens undergoes peristalsis, ejecting about 0.5 mL of fluid containing its store of sperms;
- the seminal vesicles expel their contents, flushing the semen out along the urethra; and
- the bulbospongiosus muscles contract repeatedly to squirt the semen out from the bulbar urethra.

Erectile impotence

Unrealistic expectations

Some men consult the doctor because they feel their performance is below par, e.g. if they cannot ejaculate more than three times per night. Age brings a normal diminution in sexual activity.

Wrong partner

Some patients can ejaculate perfectly well in their dreams or on masturbation and with one partner but not another. This is a psychological minefield where expert counselling is essential.

No desire

Many patients wake with an erection in the morning, but with no desire for intercourse. Sometimes this is a feature of overwork: frustration, alcohol and divorce are common features of the syndrome. A holiday may cure the condition, but expert counselling may be needed.

No erection at all

There are a number of organic causes for malfunction of the physiology of erection:

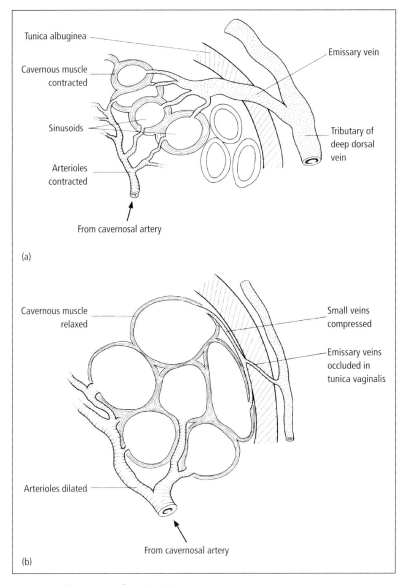

(a)

(b)

Figure 21.5 Mechanism of erection: (a) flaccid and (b) erect.

- arterial obstruction (diabetes and arteriosclerosis);
- parasympathetic disorders (diabetes, Shy–Drager syndrome);
- damage to the autonomic nerves from trauma or surgery in the pelvis; and
- medication especially with antidepressant drugs.

Investigation

The investigation of organic impotence should proceed in logical steps. Diabetes is easily excluded. The recent introduction of oral selective inhibitors of phosphodiesterase-5 (PDE-5) such as *sildenafil* has made a major impact on the investigations of erectile dysfunction. It is

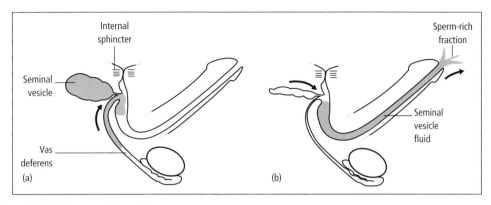

Figure 21.6 Mechanism of ejaculation.

easier to test the patient's response to one of these PDE-5 inhibitors before embarking on other investigations.

Obstruction to the blood supply of the penis can be tested by Doppler studies of the penile blood flow or by a test injection into the corpus cavernosum of one of the substances that mimics parasympathetic stimulation, e.g. papaverine or prostaglandin E. Nocturnal tumescence, which accompanies dreaming in the phase of sleep marked by rapid eye movements, can be monitored by means of paper strips (Fig. 21.7) or an electronic device (Fig. 21.8). Failure of the occlusion of the penile veins during the third, rigid phase of erection – venous leakage – can be diagnosed by injecting contrast into the corpora cavernosa and monitoring the pressure while an artificial erection is produced by the injection of prostaglandin (Fig. 21.9).

Treatment

• *Drugs: Sildenafil* may be taken by mouth up to 30–40 minutes before intercourse. It is contraindicated in men with myocardial insufficiency and care is warranted in hypertensive patients. *Yohimbine* is an alkaloid similar to reserpine, and may in some cases restore erection if given as 5 mg three times per day.
• *Vacuum devices:* These are available which suck blood into the penis to produce an artificial tumescence which is then maintained with a rubber band around the base of the penis. Many patients find this satisfactory.

• *Self-injection:* If a test injection of prostaglandin E produces a successful erection, the patient can be taught to do it himself. It is essential that he knows whom to telephone if the erection fails to subside after 3 or 4 hours so that the condition can be promptly corrected (see *priapism*).

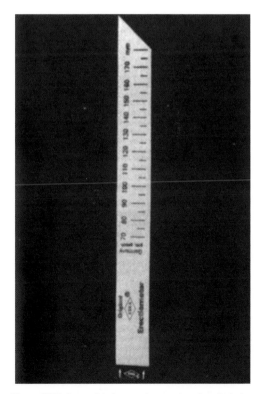

Figure 21.7 Paper strip to record expansion of penis during sleep.

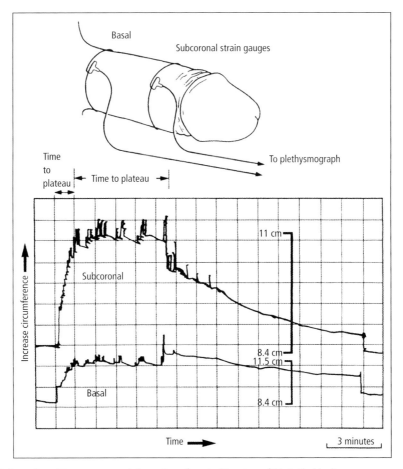

Figure 21.8 Recording of tumescence and elongation of penis. (Courtesy of Mr P. Blacklay.)

• *Implanted penile prostheses:* Devices are available which can be inserted into the corpora cavernosa to stiffen them. Some can be bent and made to straighten out, others are inflated from a concealed reservoir (Fig. 21.10). They are all expensive, and their insertion calls for great care. Being a mechanical foreign body, there is a risk of infection, erosion and mechanical failure.

• *Vascular operations:* Arterial insufficiency: attempts to improve arterial blood flow in selected patients have been tried, e.g. the inferior epigastric artery is anastomosed to the dorsal artery of the penis. Venous insufficiency: the objective is to prevent blood leaking out of the penis when a venous leak has been demonstrated.

Ejaculatory failure

Premature ejaculation

The problem here is a trigger that is too sensitive: it is not physiologically abnormal. Counselling may help, but the most simple remedy is to let the couple have a rest and try again at some convenient later time.

Inhibited ejaculation

Guilt, anxiety, a squeaky bed, fear of discovery – most young lovers and all novelists know how such factors can inhibit lovemaking. A counsellor may help.

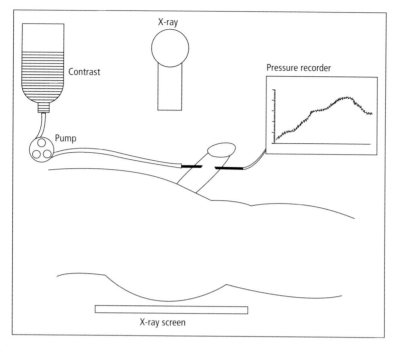

Figure 21.9 Corpus cavernosography.

No ejaculation

1 The seminal tract may be blocked at the ejaculatory ducts. Ejaculation may be painful. Transrectal ultrasound may reveal distended seminal vesicles. It may be possible to unblock the ejaculatory ducts by incision or resection of their openings on the verumontanum.

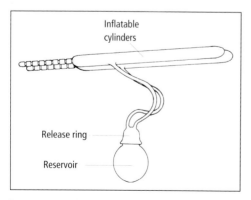

Figure 21.10 Inflatable penile prosthesis. (Surgitek Uni-flate 1000.)

2 A urethral stricture may prevent the escape of semen.

3 Retrograde ejaculation may be taking place because of previous surgery at the bladder neck, or because the sympathetic innervation of the bladder neck has been destroyed by trauma or surgery in the pelvis, or by medication with an alpha-blocker. A sympathomimetic drug, e.g. ephedrine may cure the problem.

Priapism

In priapism the corpora cavernosa are rigid, but the glans penis is soft. There are two types of priapism:
• *Low-flow priapism:* This may occur after normal intercourse, after medication with alpha-blocking drugs such as prazosin, in certain haematological conditions such as sickle-cell disease and leukaemia, and in patients undergoing haemodialysis. It is most often seen after self-injection with papaverine or prostaglandin E for impotence.
• *High-flow priapism:* This is rare, and occurs when injury has led to an aneurysm of the deep artery of

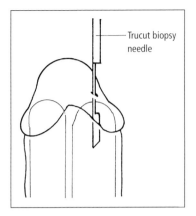

Figure 21.11 Hole made between glans penis and corpus cavernosum with biopsy needle.

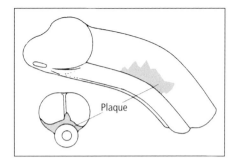

Figure 21.12 Peyronie's disease.

the corpus cavernosum. A Doppler study will show the high blood flow and measurement of the pO$_2$ of blood aspirated from the penis will show that it resembles arterial blood.

Treatment

Low-flow priapism when seen in leukaemia and dialysis, requires no treatment other than bed rest and analgesia. In sickle-cell disease plasmapheresis can be used to rid the blood of misshapen red cells. In the other more common forms of priapism an intracavernosal injection of *noradrenaline* or *aramine* is given and usually rapidly reverses the process. If this fails, a hole is made between the flaccid glans penis or corpus spongiosum and the rigid corpora cavernosa either with a biopsy needle (Fig. 21.11) or by surgical anastomosis. The treatment is urgent because delay may be followed by irreversible changes in the lining of the sinuses of the spongy tissue of the corpora which may lead to permanent erectile impotence.

In high-flow priapism selective angiography and embolisation may produce a cure.

Peyronie's disease

Plaques of fibrous tissue develop in Buck's fascia or the septum between the corpora cavernosa (Fig. 21.12). During an erection the part affected by fibrosis does not fill so the penis bends over. The cause is not known. It may occur in association with similar lumps of fibrous tissue in the palms of the hands (Dupuytren's contracture), nodules in the ears and retroperitoneal fibrosis.

The treatment of Peyronie's disease offers rich pickings to the quack: everything from acupuncture to radiotherapy has been used. Potaba (potassium amino benzoate) is thought to be efficacious but is poorly tolerated by some patients and is costly. Vitamin E is thought to be effective and is safe and inexpensive. The latest in a long line of medications is *tamoxifen*, which is said to be promising. Whatever treatment is given, in many cases the discomfort ceases and the deformity reduces spontaneously. Large lumps of fibrous tissue disappear. Frequently all that the patient needs is reassurance. Recent attempts at shock waves fragmentation of hard, nearly calcified plaques, are being evaluated.

When the condition is particularly painful, or the angulation of the penis prevents intercourse, the penis can be straightened by taking a series of tucks in the tunica on the side opposite to the plaque (Fig. 21.13). The patient should be made aware that some loss of penile shaft length can occur. Excision of the plaques and tissue replacement (dermal grafts or venous patches) has been considered. A penile prosthesis can be offered in more advanced cases.

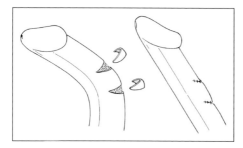

Figure 21.13 Correction of the curvature in Peyronie's disease.

Inflammation of the penis

Acute balanitis

Acute balanitis occurs in men who cannot retract the foreskin to keep the preputial space and glans penis clean. It can be due to a specific infection, e.g. *Haemophilus ducreyii*, which causes chancroid, and *Candida albicans*, which occurs particularly commonly in diabetic men. Recurrent acute balanitis is one indication for therapeutic circumcision.

Ulceration on the glans penis may be due to primary infection with syphilis, in which case the spirochaetes of *Treponema pallidum* can be identified in the serum which is expressed from the ulcer. Its diagnosis and treatment is a matter for the appropriate experts to whom the patient should be referred.

Cancer of the penis

Aetiology

Cancer of the penis occurs in uncircumcised men who are usually old and unwashed and whose foreskin has never been pulled back to keep the glans clean.

There has been endless debate over the issue of preventing cancer of the penis by routine neonatal circumcision. Childhood circumcision certainly does prevent cancer of the penis, but has its own mortality and morbidity, and it has been calcu-

lated that slightly more deaths would occur if all boys were to be circumcised than would occur from cancer of the penis, at least in the West. Soap and water appear to be just as effective in preventing penile cancer.

Other known predisposing factors are smoking, papillomavirus infections and previous recurrent balanitis. There are also four well-recognised precancerous conditions:

• *Erythroplasia of Queyrat:* This is a form of carcinoma in situ of the skin of the glans. It resembles balanitis, and is diagnosed by means of a biopsy. It can be cured with local coagulation with a CO_2 laser, or 5-fluorouracil cream. If neglected it progresses to overt cancer (Fig. 21.14).

• *Balanitis xerotica obliterans:* This is a skin condition, identical with lichen sclerosus et obliterans. It is common, and usually benign, but may proceed to cancer and should always be followed up. There is a whitish alteration in the skin of the prepuce causing it to become stiff, tight and difficult to retract. When the condition affects the glans penis it produces a stenosis of the external urinary meatus which may require surgical correction (Fig. 21.15).

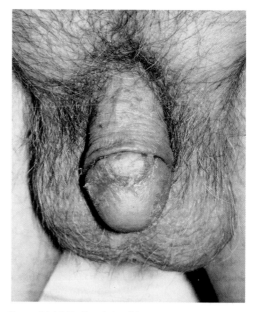

Figure 21.14 Erythroplasia of Queyrat.

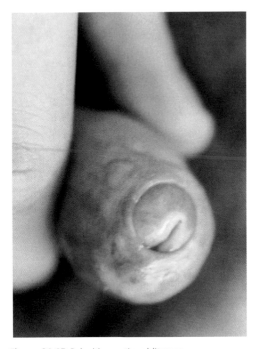

Figure 21.15 Balanitis xerotica obliterans.

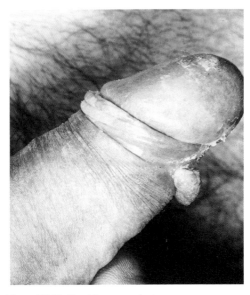

Figure 21.16 Condyloma acuminatum.

- *Condyloma acuminatum:* This is a benign wart caused by one of the family of papilloma viruses (Fig. 21.16). It responds to local measures such as podophyllin, freezing and diathermy.
- *Giant condyloma acuminatum:* It is sometimes seen in a giant form, the *Buschke–Löwenstein tumour*. At first this contains papilloma virus and seems histologically to be benign, but if not treated radically always progresses to invasive cancer.

Pathology

Cancer of the penis occurs in three macroscopic forms, an ulcer, a papilliferous cauliflower or a nodule (Fig. 21.17). There is always secondary infection, and many of these cases present late in the course of the disease with a profuse, evil-smelling discharge from beneath an inflamed prepuce. The inguinal lymph nodes are often enlarged because of infection.

Grade

These are all squamous cell cancers. There are three histological grades of tumour, G1–G3, according to the frequency of mitoses that are present (Fig. 21.18).

Stage grouping (see Fig. 21.19)

Stage I: Tumour confined to glans penis, prepuce or both.

Stage II: Tumour involves penile shaft or corpora; negative nodes.

Stage III: Tumour confined to penis with operable inguinal lymph node metastases.

Stage IV: Tumour extends beyond penile shaft with inoperable inguinal or distant lymph nodes, or distant metastases.

TNM classification

T – Primary tumour:

Tis: cancer in situ

Ta: non-invasive verrucous carcinoma

T1: tumour invades subepithelia connective tissue

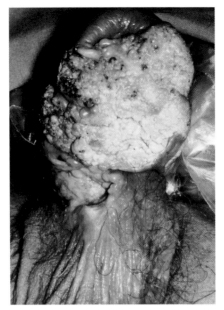
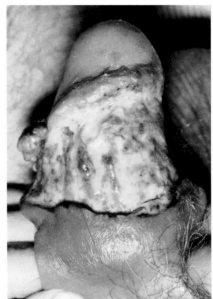

Figure 21.17 Papillary and ulcerated types of carcinoma of the penis.

T2: tumour invades corporal body

T3: tumour invades urethra or prostate

T4: tumour invades other adjacent structures

N – Regional lymph nodes:

Nx: not assessed

N0: no regional lymph node metastases

N1: a single superficial lymph node metastases

N2: multiple or bilateral superficial lymph node metastases

N3: deep inguinal or pelvic lymph node metastases, unilateral or bilateral

M – Distant metastases:

Mx: not assessed

M0: no distant metastases

M1: distant metastases present

Diagnosis

At first the diagnosis is in doubt, and the first step is a circumcision to uncover the tumour

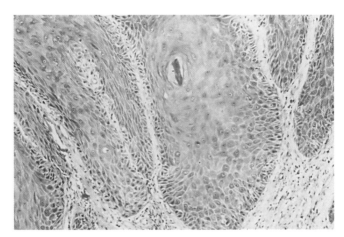

Figure 21.18 Squamous cell carcinoma of penis. (Courtesy of Professor Jo Martin.)

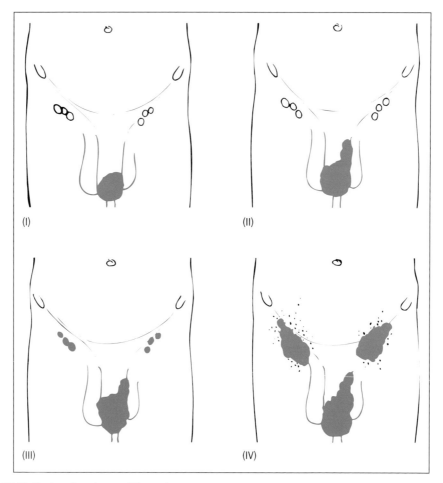

Figure 21.19 Staging of carcinoma of the penis.

and obtain a biopsy. At this stage there is usually much secondary infection and the inguinal lymph nodes are often enlarged because of inflammation.

Treatment

Stage I

If not entirely removed by circumcision, the choice of treatment is partial amputation (Fig. 21.20) or local radiotherapy. Both can produce 100% cure but after radiotherapy there is a 20% chance of local recurrence that eventually requires partial amputation.

Stage II

Local radiation still offers 100% cure, but 50% will require partial amputation for residual or recurrent disease. Preliminary radiation improves the long-term survival. It is important to know that even after partial amputation patients can still enjoy a normal sex life.

Stage III

If the scrotum is involved, wide radical excision offers an excellent chance of cure.

Stage IV

When the inguinal nodes are involved, as may be shown by cytological examination of fluid

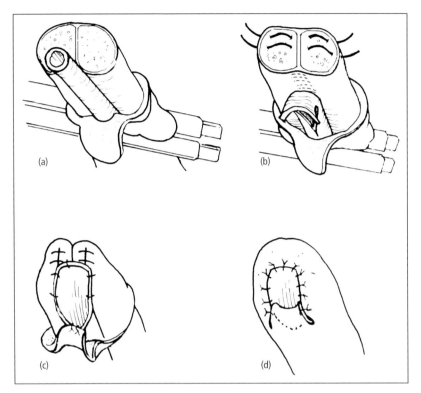

Figure 21.20 Partial amputation of the penis.

aspirated from an inguinal node, computed tomography scanning is performed to detect involvement of nodes along the iliac vessels and aorta. Treatment is by a combination of chemotherapy and block dissection of all the nodes that are found to be involved. The major complication of block dissection of the inguinal lymph nodes is distressing oedema of the lower limb, which can only in part be prevented or relieved by supportive stockings.

Chapter 22

The testicle

Embryology

The germ cells arise in the yolk sac of the foetus, migrate along the umbilical cord, and bury themselves in the urogenital gonadal ridge on the back of the coelom (Fig. 22.1). Later the future testis bulges forwards, and then follows a lump of jelly called the *gubernaculum* downwards into the scrotum, carrying with it a bag of peritoneum in front

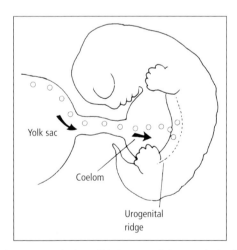

Figure 22.1 The incredible journey of the germinal cells from the yolk sac to the urogenital ridge.

Yolk sac

Coelom

Urogenital ridge

Lecture Notes: Urology, 6th edition. By John Blandy and Amir Kaisary. Published 2009 by Blackwell Publishing. ISBN: 978-1-4051-2270-2.

and reaching the scrotum shortly before birth (Fig. 22.2).

Surgical anatomy

The term *testicle* includes both testis and epididymis. The testis lies in front of the epididymis, slung from the external inguinal ring by the spermatic cord. In front of the testis and nearly surrounding it is the tunica vaginalis, remnant of the peritoneum. It contains only a trace of fluid.

Blood supply

The testicular artery arises from the aorta near the renal arteries and passes in front of the ureter and curls round lateral to the inferior epigastric vessels to enter the inguinal canal. The numerous large veins which drain the testicle form the *pampiniform plexus* which join together to enter the vena cava on the right and the renal vein on the left (Fig. 22.3).

Structure

Testis

Each testis is made up of sets of tubules arranged in loops, which empty into a sac, the rete testis. This drains through a dozen *vasa efferentia* into the

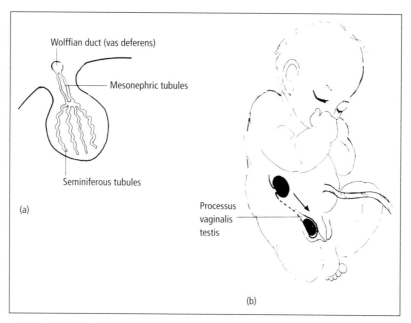

(a)

(b)

Figure 22.2 Normal descent of the testicle.

epididymis (Fig. 22.4). The testicular tubule contains two types of cell – germinal cells and Sertoli cells. In between them there is a packing of Leydig cells (Fig. 22.5).

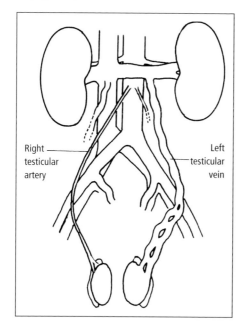

Figure 22.3 Blood supply of the testicle.

The *germinal* cells divide into successive generations of spermatocytes which ultimately develop by mitosis and meiosis into spermatozoa (Fig. 22.6).

The Sertoli cells secrete *inhibin* which regulates the pituitary supply of luteinizing hormone (Fig. 22.7).

The Leydig cells secrete *testosterone*.

Epididymis

The epididymis is a long coiled tube lying behind the testis, which continues as the vas deferens. It is lined with microcilia similar to those in the bronchioles (Fig. 22.8).

Vas deferens

The vas deferens runs along the back of the spermatic cord, curls around the inferior epigastric vessels, crosses in front of the ureter and passes in the cleft between the inner and outer zones of the prostate to join the common ejaculatory duct and open into the prostatic urethra on the

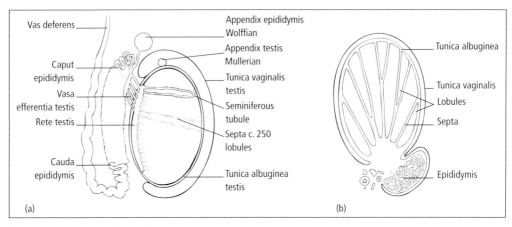

Figure 22.4 Structure of the testicle.

verumontanum. The vas deferens has a powerful muscular wall, and is lined with columnar epithelium. It acts as a reservoir for sperms, emptying on ejaculation (Fig. 22.9).

Seminal vesicle

The seminal vesicle lies behind the prostate, just under the bladder. It is a long duct, coiled up so that on cross-section it resembles a honeycomb.

Its duct joins the vas deferens to form the *common ejaculatory duct* (Fig. 22.10).

Congenital anomalies of the testicle

Undescended testicle

There are two kinds of undescended testicle, those in which the gubernaculum has gone off

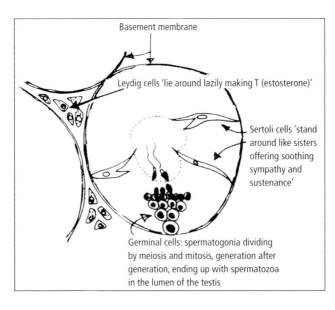

Figure 22.5 Diagram of testicular tubule.

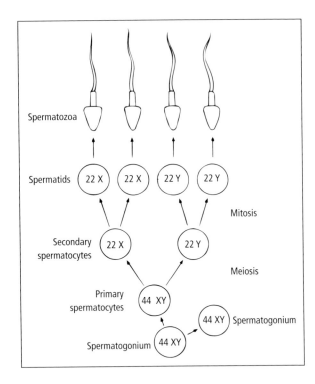

Figure 22.6 Spermatogenesis.

course – ectopic – and those in which the descent to the bottom of the scrotum is incomplete – incomplete descent (Fig. 22.11).

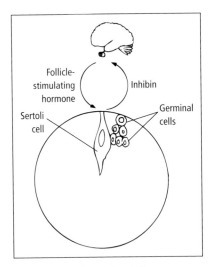

Figure 22.7 Sertoli cells and the pituitary.

Ectopic testicle

The errant gubernaculum may guide the ectopic testicle into one of four positions:

> *inguinal*, in the abdominal wall near the external inguinal ring;
> *perineal*;
> *penile*, near the base of the penis; and
> *crural*, in the thigh (Fig. 22.12).

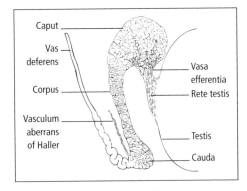

Figure 22.8 Anatomy of the epididymis.

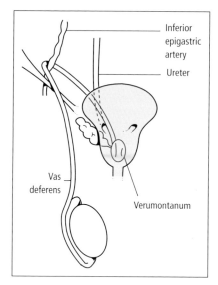

Figure 22.9 Surgical anatomy of the vas deferens.

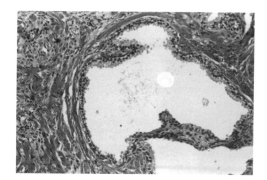

Figure 22.10 Histology of seminal vesicle.

Incomplete descent

The testicles always move up and down, and are defined according to their range of movement as:

• *abdominal*, which may move in and out of the internal inguinal ring;

• *inguinal*, which move along the inguinal canal;

• *emergent*, when they appear at the external ring;

• *high retractile*, when they move up and down but cannot be made to go to the bottom of the scrotum; and

• *low retractile*, when they descend to the bottom of the scrotum in a warm bath, under general anaesthesia, or with gentle persuasion by a doctor's warm hand. Low retractile testes are essentially normal, and will always end up in the scrotum with puberty.

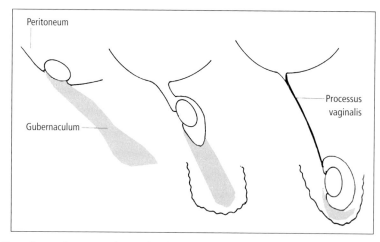

Figure 22.11 The gubernaculum opens the way for the testicle to follow into the scrotum.

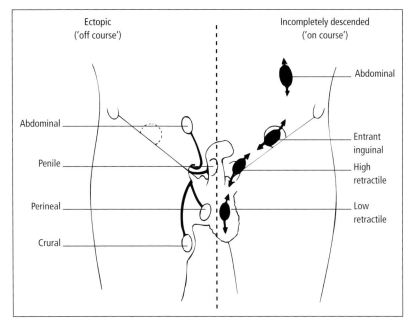

Figure 22.12 Undescended testicles may be off or on course.

Complications

1 *Torsion:* There is often a large loose sac of peritoneum in front of an emergent or retractile undescended testicle which makes it prone to torsion (see below) (Fig. 22.13).

2 *Infertility:* It is common with bilateral undescended testicles, but not with unilateral undescent.

3 *Cancer:* About 1 in 10 testicular tumours is associated with maldescent.

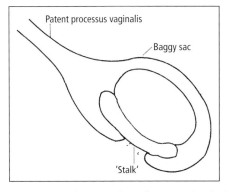

Figure 22.13 The baggy peritoneal sac associated with incomplete descent favours torsion.

Diagnosis

In most cases the diagnosis is made by inspection and palpation. Difficulty may arise with the low retractile testis: seldom is this difficult for an experienced doctor with warm hands, and a child who is not frightened. When in doubt the child should be examined in a warm bath, and if there is still doubt he may be given a general anaesthetic to see if the testicle descends to the bottom of the scrotum.

When no testicle can be felt on one side, it is often in the inguinal canal. The testicle is easily found with a computed tomography (CT) scan, even in the abdomen.

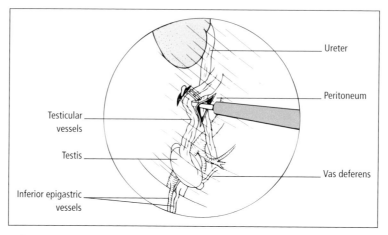

Figure 22.14 The first step in the Fowler–Stephens procedure: the testicular vessels are clipped laparoscopically.

Management

Ectopic testes

These never find their way into the scrotum and require orchiopexy.

Incomplete descent

1 *Abdominal:* These are now located by CT scan, if necessary confirmed by laparoscopy. In prepubertal boys an effort should be made to preserve the testis. In the Fowler–Stephens procedure the testicular artery is divided as a first step which may be performed through a laparoscope (Fig. 22.14). Some 6 months later at a second operation the testicle is mobilised and brought down into the scrotum, by which time it will have acquired a new blood supply from the artery to the vas (Fig. 22.15) and it is safe to divide the testicular vessels.

2 *Inguinal:* Most of these are brought down by the routine operation of orchiopexy.

Through a crease incision over the internal ring, the external oblique is opened, the testicle is mobilized, taking care not to injure its artery or the vas deferens. The testicular vessels are followed up behind the peritoneum and mobilised medially by dividing fibrous bands. This allows the testicle to be placed in a sac between the dartos

muscle and skin of the scrotum without tension (Fig. 22.16).

Timing of orchiopexy. Although 90% of testicles are in the scrotum at birth, the next 9% do not descend until 12 months, after which no more do. Infertility, and possibly the late development of cancer, is thought to be prevented by orchiopexy performed before the age of 3, so there is a window of opportunity between ages 2 and 3, but at this age the technique is difficult. The best results are only obtained in specialised paediatric centres.

After puberty the chance of improving fertility is minimal, and the risk of cancer increases rapidly, but most young men wish to keep both testes.

When an undescended testicle is found in a mature grown man, orchiectomy is the procedure that should be advised in view of the risks of malignancy. If the patient is concerned about his cosmetic appearance he may be offered a silicone prosthesis.

Hormone treatment. Puberty can be brought on early by giving pituitary gonadotrophins, which accelerate the descent of a low retractile testis but at the price of premature puberty and stunting of growth from early fusion of epiphyses. The method is no longer used.

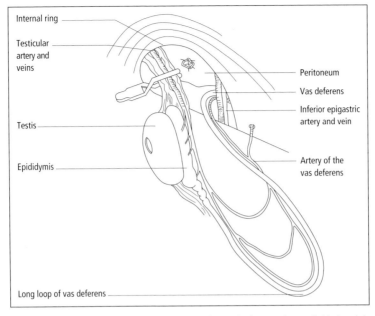

Figure 22.15 Second stage in the Fowler–Stephens procedure: the testicular vessels are divided and the testicle brought down.

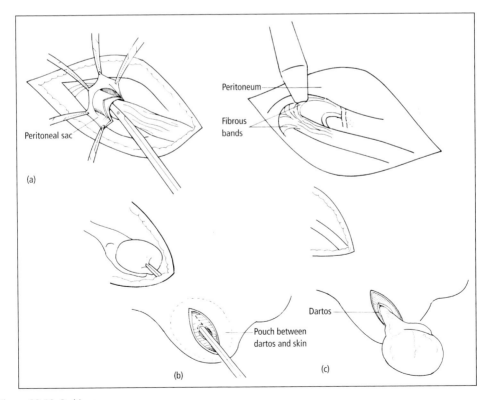

Figure 22.16 Orchiopexy.

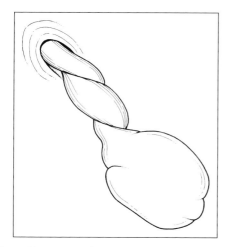

Figure 22.17 Neonatal extravaginal torsion.

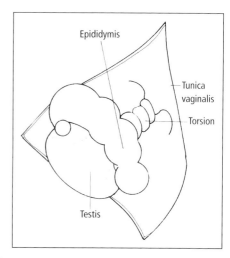

Figure 22.18 Intravaginal torsion of the testicle.

Torsion

Extravaginal

This is rarely seen in newborn boys. The testicle has rotated on the spermatic cord and it is almost never possible to save the testis by untwisting it (Fig. 22.17).

Intravaginal

The tunica vaginalis may be unusually roomy even with a normally descended testicle, and the testis and epididymis can twist on a stalk like a light-bulb in its socket (Fig. 22.18). Patients often re-call attacks of pain that come on and are relieved equally suddenly, and a history of such warning attacks is sufficient reason to explore the testicle and fix it.

Torsion may occur at any age, but is most common around puberty.

Clinical features

There is a sudden onset of pain and swelling in the testicle which may wake the boy. On examination the scrotum is tender, red and swollen, and it is seldom possible to make out testis from epididymis (Fig. 22.19).

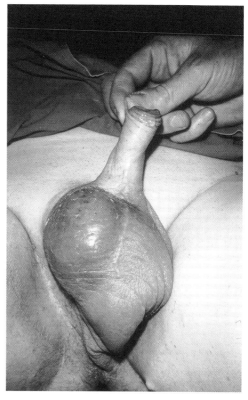

Figure 22.19 Appearance of torsion of the testicle.

The differential diagnosis is from:

1 *mumps orchitis*, which never attacks boys before puberty;

2 *epididymitis*, which is always secondary to obvious urinary infection;

3 *fat necrosis*, which is occasionally seen in infants;

4 *cancer*, which in older boys and men can present with inflammation; and

5 *torsion of an appendix testis*, which cannot be distinguished from torsion of the testis without exploration.

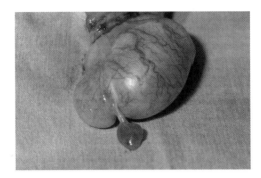

Figure 22.20 Torsion of an appendix testis.

Investigations

It is important to untwist the testicle before it dies from ischaemia, and no investigation should be allowed to delay surgical exploration. A Doppler or radioisotope scan may show absence of arterial circulation in the testicle but is justified only if it will not delay matters.

Treatment

The testicle is explored through a transverse scrotal incision. The tunica vaginalis is opened, and the testicle is untwisted. If there is any doubt about the viability of the testis it can be incised to see if it still bleeds. All too often it is necrotic and must be removed.

Because torsion occurs in about 10% of cases on the other side, the other testicle should be fixed then or at a later operation.

Torsion of the appendix testis

Tiny cysts are usually present at the upper pole, one on the epididymis (Wolffian duct origin), the other on the testis (Müllerian duct origin). Apart from being of interest to embryologists either can twist on its stalk, exactly mimicking torsion of the testicle and equally requiring urgent exploration (Fig. 22.20).

Varicocele

The normal pampiniform plexus of veins draining the testicle has been thought to act as a heat-exchanger to keep the testicle cool. A varicocele is a physiological dilatation of these veins (Fig. 22.21). It is widely believed to depress spermatogenesis and lead to atrophy of the testis, and many operations are performed for this reason although every controlled study so far has shown that the operations make no difference. The testicular vessels are approached through a short incision above and parallel to the inguinal ligament, the veins are separated from the testicular artery, ligated and divided. It has become fashionable to do the same thing via a laparoscope.

Hydrocele

Fluid accumulates in the cavity of the tunica vaginalis testis. These may be primary or idiopathic (i.e. there is no obvious cause), or they may be secondary to obstruction to the lymphatic drainage of the testicle, or part of widespread oedema caused by heart failure, or as an inflammatory effusion from underlying disease in the testis or epididymis (Fig. 22.22). The swelling is fluctuant and a light shines easily through it.

Neonatal

When a hydrocele in a neonate is associated with a hernia, it is operated on almost as an emergency in view of the risk of strangulation. The processus vaginalis is found at the external ring and ligated. There is no need to do anything about the tunica vaginalis testis (Fig. 22.23).

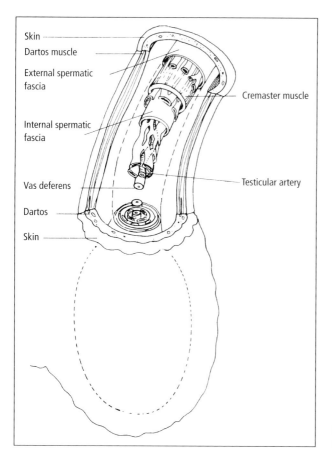

Skin

Dartos muscle

External spermatic fascia

Internal spermatic fascia

Vas deferens

Dartos

Skin

Cremaster muscle

Testicular artery

Figure 22.21 The veins of the spermatic cord.

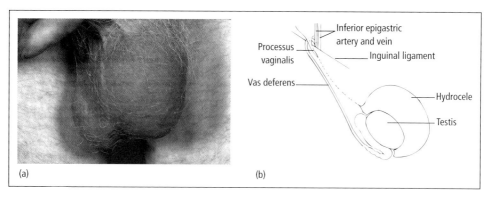

Inferior epigastric artery and vein

Processus vaginalis

Inguinal ligament

Vas deferens

Hydrocele

Testis

(a)

(b)

Figure 22.22 Hydrocele: (a) clinical presentation and (b) diagram.

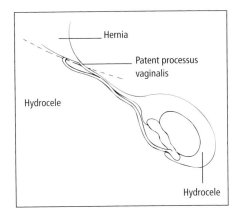

Figure 22.23 Infantile hydrocele.

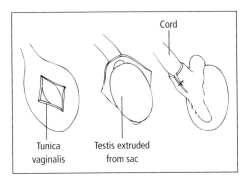

Figure 22.25 Jaboulay operation for hydrocele.

Adult

In an adult there is always a suspicion that that the hydrocele may be concealing some mischief in the testis. Ultrasound screening is performed to ensure that the underlying testis is healthy, and if there is any doubt, tumour markers are measured to rule out cancer of the testis.

Few hydroceles need any treatment: a good rule is to offer an operation if the patient's wife or his tailor complains. The options are to aspirate the fluid (Fig. 22.24), warning the patient that it will fill up again, or remove the surplus tunica vaginalis (Fig. 22.25).

Cysts of the epididymis

A few tiny cysts are always present in the upper end of the epididymis, arising as diverticula of the vasa efferentia and epididymal tubules. In middle age a few pea-sized cysts can usually be felt. Occasionally these cysts become large enough to be a nuisance.

The swellings are always fluctuant and usually transmit light easily. If aspirated, the fluid may look opalescent, like lime water, because a few sperms are present. Occasionally there are so many to make the fluid look like cream. Pregnancy has been reported by injecting these sperms.

The diagnosis is easily confirmed by ultrasound. Treatment is seldom necessary. Aspiration is usually futile because the cysts fill up again and they are always multilocular. Excision of the cysts often results in a blockage of the vasa efferentia, and should be postponed until the patient has completed his family (Figs. 22.26 and 22.27).

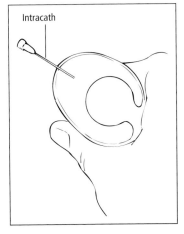

Figure 22.24 Tapping a hydrocele.

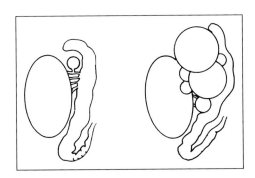

Figure 22.26 Cysts of the epididymis (a diagram).

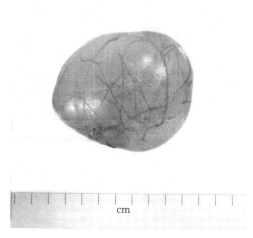

Figure 22.27 An epididymal cyst (a photograph).

Trauma to the testicle

The testis is easily injured in sport or at work. Blood collects in the cavity of the tunica vaginalis. The danger is that expansion of the clot may produce pressure-atrophy of the rest of the testis, and for this reason injured testes should all be explored, the clot evacuated, and the rent in the tunica albuginea sewn up (Fig. 22.28).

Testicular tumours are notoriously apt to present after trauma and surgeons must always keep this possibility in mind because an orchiectomy may be needed.

Inflammation of the testicle

Acute orchitis

Most infections in the testis are caused by viruses, e.g. Coxsackie or mumps. *Mumps orchitis* only occurs after puberty, when it may be bilateral and the oedema may lead to pressure necrosis and atrophy of the testis. When unilateral it may be impossible to distinguish from torsion and therefore demands to be explored. There is some evidence that incision of the *tunica albuginea* will decompress the testis and prevent atrophy.

Acute epididymitis

Bacterial infection finds its way down the vas deferens from the urinary tract to cause acute inflammation. This is seen after operations on the urinary tract especially if a catheter has been left in the urethra. The organisms are usually *Escherichia coli*. Acute epididymitis arising out of the blue may be caused by *Chlamydia trachomatis*, which can be identified in fluid aspirated from the epididymis with special culture techniques. Rarely, tuberculosis can cause surprisingly acute symptoms and should be excluded in every acute case where there is no obvious cause for infection such as a recent operation on the urinary tract.

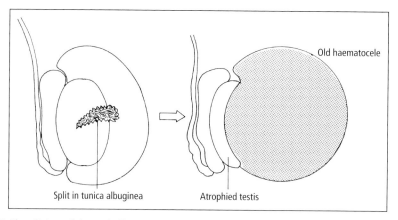

Figure 22.28 Closed injury of the testis: if not evacuated, the clot may cause atrophy of the testis.

Chronic orchitis

Syphilitic gumma of the testis was for a generation only a pathological curiosity. Cancer is far more likely and in any event, orchiectomy is probably the right treatment.

Granulomatous orchitis occurs with repeated urinary infections and does not always respond to antibiotics, and usually requires orchiectomy.

Chronic epididymitis

Tuberculosis

Blood-borne infection with *Mycobacterium tuberculosis* occurs in the head of the epididymis: urine-borne infection involves the tail along with the vas deferens (Fig. 22.29). The epididymis is knobbly and hard, and there may be nodules along the vas. In late cases a sinus may form and discharge on the skin of the scrotum. Rectal ultrasound scanning may show tuberculosis of the prostate and seminal vesicles. The diagnosis and treatment follow the rules for tuberculosis elsewhere. After a full course of treatment a residual mass in the epididymis may have to be removed.

Seminal granuloma

After vasectomy many men have induration in the epididymis caused by an inflammatory response

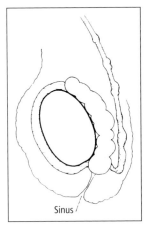

Figure 22.29 Tuberculosis of the epididymis and vas deferens.

to extravasated sperms. It may respond to prednisolone.

Orchialgia

There is a sad group of men who complain of persistent pain in the testicle. Often there has been some previous minor surgical operation, e.g. vasectomy or hydrocelectomy, and pain persists. Careful clinical examination can find nothing wrong. An ultrasound scan is normal. Frequently the testicle is explored and nothing abnormal can be found. Before long the patient seeks a second opinion, and almost inevitably another surgeon will attempt to denervate the testicle. The result is instant relief of pain – for a while, but then it comes back.

Before long the patient has persuaded yet another surgeon to remove the testicle. This is done: once again the relief of pain is dramatic – for a while, and then it comes back on the other side. It is most important to recognise these unfortunate men because they need help, but from the psychiatrist not the surgeon.

Cancer of the testis

Aetiology

Although there are only about 500 new cases in the UK per annum (about 4.5 per 100,000 males), it is the most common cancer in men under the age of 35. It is rare in men of African ancestry both in Africa and elsewhere. It is rare before puberty, and peaks in the early twenties.

One in 10 tumours occurs in association with maldescent of the testis.

Pathology

Cancer may arise from any of the cell types present in the testis; over 90% arise from germ cells (Fig. 22.30).

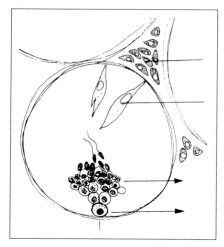

Figure 22.30 Cellular origin of testicular tumours.

Germ cell tumours

Gonadocytes and spermatocytes

These give rise to a spectrum of tumours, from highly anaplastic seminoma which shows nuclear polymorphism and may even stain for human chorionic gonadotrophin, through intermediate types with sheets of cells filled with glycogen that stain for placental alkaline phosphatase (PLAP), to well-differentiated spermatocytic seminoma which seldom metastasize (Figs. 22.31 and 23.32).

Embryonal carcinoma

Here the tissues attempt to form organs, with papillary and glandular elements. They stain for alpha-foetoprotein (AFP) which betrays the origin of germ cells from the foetal yolk-sac. Pure

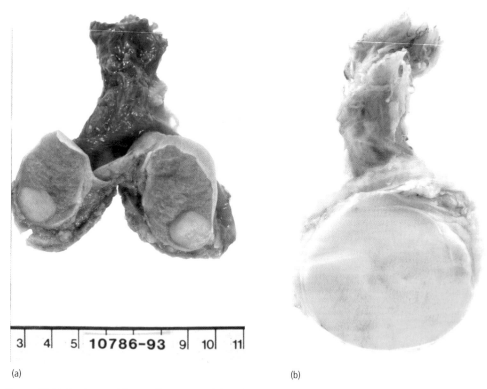

(a)

(b)

Figure 22.31 Seminoma: (a) a small tumour nodule within the testis and (b) a tumour replacing all normal testicular tissue.

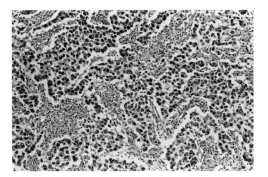

Figure 22.32 Seminoma: microscopic appearance.

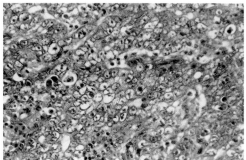

Figure 22.34 Teratocarcinoma: macroscopic appearance.

yolk-sac tumours are occasionally found in infants (Fig. 22.33).

Epidermoid cyst

A cyst containing mature tissue, mainly skin, is occasionally found. Some of them are possibly be-nign, but it can take very careful histological ex-amination to distinguish it from teratocarcinoma.

Teratocarcinoma

In this there is a spectrum from the most benign-looking adult tissues, e.g. cartilage and hair, to wildly malignant choriocarcinoma. Of all the pos-sibilities, choriocarcinoma is the worst, spreading rapidly through the bloodstream (Figs. 22.34 and 22.35).

Non-germ cell tumours

Leydig cell tumours

These arise from the Leydig cells that are packed in between the tubules of the testis and normally pro-duce testosterone. They can give rise to precocious puberty.

Sertoli cell tumours

These are very rare, seldom metastasize and cause gynaecomastia.

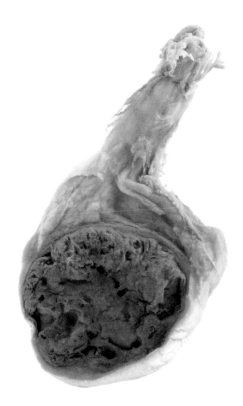

Figure 22.33 Embryonal carcinoma.

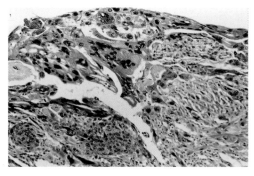

Figure 22.35 Teratocarcinoma: microscopic appearance.

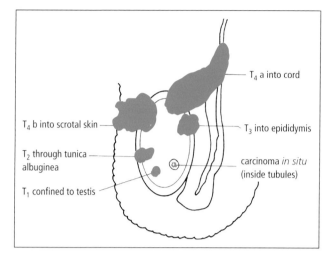

Figure 22.36 T staging of testis tumours.

Lymphomas

They may be confined to the testis, and tend to occur in older men.

TNM staging of testicular tumours

T stage

The T stage is determined only after careful histological examination of the entire testicle (Fig. 22.36).

N stage

The testis drains to the para-aortic lymph nodes at the level of the origin of the renal arteries, and only later via the cisterna chyli into the thoracic duct and systemic circulation. The nodes are localised by CT scanning (Fig. 22.37).

M stage

Venous spread can occur early if trophoblastic elements are present.

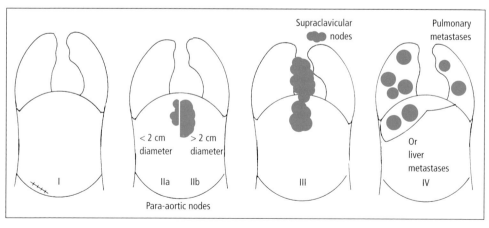

Figure 22.37 N staging of testis tumours (Royal Marsden Hospital system).

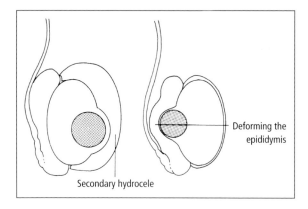

Secondary hydrocele

Deforming the epididymis

Figure 22.38 Some testicular tumours are difficult to feel.

Clinical features

Symptoms

- *Lump in the testicle:* This is in the body of the testis. It is not fluctuant or translucent. The tragedy is that so many young men report this so late (see below).
- *'Inflammation':* About 15% have signs of inflammation that are all too easily mistaken for epididymitis.
- *Trauma:* Another 10–15% of men have a history of injury which may lead to loss of valuable time in making the proper diagnosis.
- *Gynaecomastia:* Transient swelling of the breasts is common at puberty, but can be due to trophoblastic elements secreting human chorionic gonadotrophin (HCG), which should be measured in every case.
- *Back pain:* The back pain in a fit young man should always make one think of metastases from a testicular tumour.

Physical signs

A hard lump is found in the body of the testis. Difficulty arises if the lump is near the epididymis, concealed in the body of the testis, or impossible to feel because of a tense hydrocele (Fig. 22.38). Inflammation can be misleading.

Always examine the breasts for gynaecomastia.

Investigations

- *Ultrasound scan:* This investigation is so quick and painless that it should be performed on every suspicious testicle (Fig. 22.39). Mistakes are rare.
- *Tumour markers:* Blood is sent for placental alkaline phosphatase (PLAP) which is secreted by gonadocytes, for HCG which is secreted by trophoblastic cells, and AFP secreted by yolk-sac cells. (An ordinary 'pregnancy test' is a quick and cheap way of detecting abnormal amounts of HCG.) Lactic acid dehydrogenase has low specificity (high false-positive rate) and should be correlated with other clinical findings. High levels can be detected in smooth, cardiac and skeletal muscle, liver, kidney and brain. It is thought to have a direct relationship with tumour burden, thus it seems to be most useful as a marker for tumour bulk tissue.
- *Exploration of the testicle:* The spermatic cord is clamped at the internal ring before the testicle is delivered: the diagnosis of cancer is usually obvious to the naked eye, but can be verified by frozen section if in doubt. The cord is transected above the clamp (Fig. 22.40).
- *CT scan:* A CT scan is performed of the chest and abdomen to identify lymph node and pulmonary metastases (Fig. 22.41).

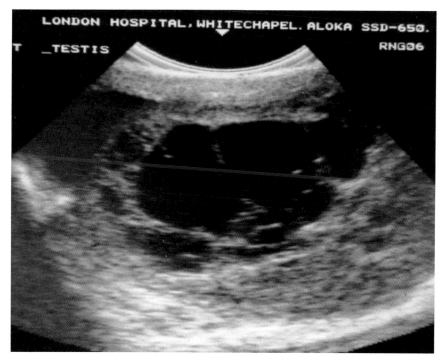

Figure 22.39 Ultrasound scan of a testicular teratoma. (Courtesy of Dr W. Hately.)

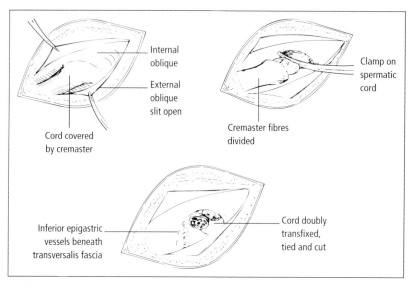

Internal
oblique

External
oblique
slit open

Cord covered
by cremaster

Clamp on
spermatic
cord

Cremaster fibres
divided

Inferior epigastric
vessels beneath
transversalis fascia

Cord doubly
transfixed,
tied and cut

Figure 22.40 Left orchiectomy.

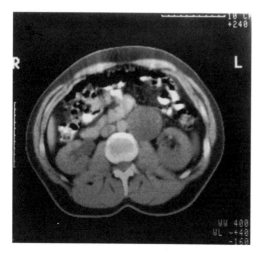

Figure 22.41 CT scan showing para-aortic mass on the left side of the aorta.

Treatment

The treatment of testicular tumours has been revolutionised by platinum-based chemotherapy. Chemotherapy is so unpleasant for the patient that attempts have been made to select out those

patients who do not need it, and follow them by surveillance. After many trials surveillance is now restricted to a small group from which excludes all seminomas, any germ cell tumours which have invaded the tissues around the testis, and any that secrete AFP or HCG.

Stage I
Staging retroperitoneal lymph node dissection
This is performed in many centres to identify microscopic metastases with the advantage that removing the lymph nodes may cure those with small volume disease. Where there are larger amounts of tumour present in the lymph nodes, chemotherapy is given afterwards. In most UK centres reliance is placed for staging on CT scanning.

Seminoma
Prophylactic radiation to the retroperitoneal lymph nodes can given 100% cure with stage I seminoma. An identical rate of cure is obtained with a single course of single-agent carboplatin. Surveillance is not an option, because of the high rate of relapse.

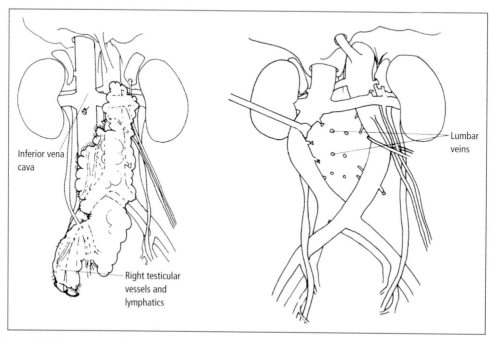

Inferior vena cava

Right testicular vessels and lymphatics

Lumbar veins

Figure 22.42 Removal of residual para-aortic nodes.

Other germ cell tumours

Surveillance is reasonable for non-seminomatous germ cell tumours without invasion of the veins or lymphatics of the testis, without yolk-sac elements, and without undifferentiated elements but because of the high rate of relapse some centres have reverted to a policy of giving all these men prophylactic platinum-based combination chemotherapy.

Stage II

All patients are given chemotherapy to start with and are then followed carefully, by serial tumour markers and CT scans.

Stage III

All patients are given as much chemotherapy as they can tolerate. If a mass remains after two or sometimes three cycles of treatment, it is removed surgically. If the mass of lymph nodes is in the retroperitoneal tissue, this requires careful dissection of all the tumours off the aorta and inferior vena cava (Fig. 22.42). Residual masses in the lungs or mediastinum are removed through the chest.

The continual advances in the management of testicular cancer have resulted in a miraculous improvement in results. In one group of 9288 patients in Southeast England between 1960 and 2004, the 10-year relative survival increased from 78% in 1960–1969 to 99% in 1990–2004 for seminomas (5555 cases), and from 55 to 95% for non-seminomas (3733 cases). This improvement is largely attributable to chemotherapy where the trend to further reducing its toxicity should continue to improve the future health of the growing numbers of survivors of testicular cancer.

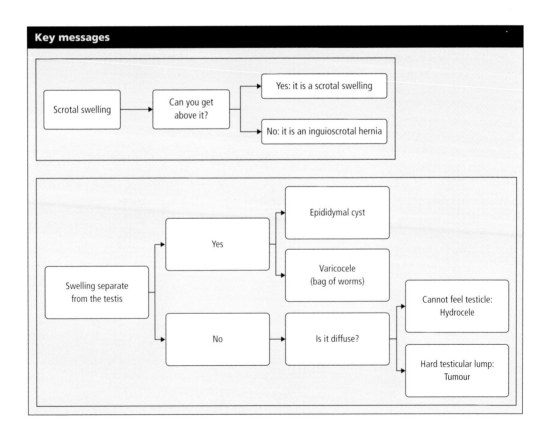

Key messages

Scrotal swelling → Can you get above it? →
- Yes: it is a scrotal swelling
- No: it is an inguioscrotal hernia

Swelling separate from the testis →
- Yes →
  - Epididymal cyst
  - Varicocele (bag of worms)
- No → Is it diffuse? →
  - Cannot feel testicle: Hydrocele
  - Hard testicular lump: Tumour

Chapter 23

Male fertility

History and general examination

Gross endocrine deficiencies are usually obvious: the young man who shaves daily and has a normal physique is unlikely to have a deficiency of androgens. Corticosteroids taken by athletes may suppress pituitary gonadotrophins. Note any history of previous surgery to the bladder neck or pelvis that may have injured the autonomic nervous system leading to probably retrograde ejaculation. Chronic illnesses such as diabetes, renal failure and liver failure can impair spermatogenesis. A past history of genitourinary infections may be relevant (e.g. mumps, gonorrhoea and non-specific urethritis). Endogenous toxins as a result of smoking and drinking alcohol could harm sperm production. Patients with recurrent sinusitis and chest infections may have epididymal obstruction (cystic fibrosis).

It is important to establish if normal ejaculation occurs within the vagina. Sexual intercourse taking place around the point of maximal female fertility (i.e. ovulation) is of prime value.

Testicles

Very small testes should raise the suspicion of Klinefelter's syndrome (XXY) (Fig. 23.1). The diag-

nosis is easily confirmed by cytology of a scraping from the mucosa of the cheek, looking for the Barr body – the index of the extra X chromosome. Note the clinical features (Table 23.1). Previous surgery for repair of a hernia, or orchidopexy, may suggest damage to the vas deferens. Previous bilateral orchidopexy often, but not always, means that both testicles are not producing sperm.

Investigations

Semen analysis (Table 23.2)

Semen is collected by masturbation after 72 hours abstinence into a clean plastic container.
- *Volume:* The normal range is from 1 to 8 mL. (The most usual cause for a low semen volume is clumsy collection of the specimen!)
- *Sperm density and motility:* Most traditional laboratory methods for measuring sperm density and motility are so inaccurate as to be useless. When the computerised Hamilton–Thorn system is used, normal fertility is found with a sperm density as low as 1×10^6 per mL provided motility is adequate.
- *Morphology:* There is very little correlation between morphological abnormalities and infertility. Many more are picked up by electron microscopy (Fig. 23.2), but are of doubtful relevance.
- *Antibodies:* Antibodies to the head and tail of the sperm may occur in blood, seminal plasma and cervical mucus. These may account for some of the

Lecture Notes: Urology, 6th edition. By John Blandy and Amir Kaisary. Published 2009 by Blackwell Publishing. ISBN: 978-1-4051-2270-2.

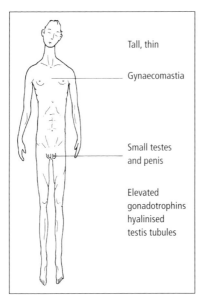

Tall, thin

Gynaecomastia

Small testes
and penis

Elevated
gonadotrophins
hyalinised
testis tubules

Figure 23.1 Klinefelter's syndrome.

immotile sperms which are sometimes found in a
post-coital test.

Luteinizing hormone and follicle-stimulating hormone measurements

A follicle-stimulating hormone (FSH) level more
than 15 mIU/mL means that the tubules are not
producing sperms, and for all practical purposes,
there is no point in doing a testicular biopsy. If
normal, it suggests that there may be a blockage
somewhere between the testis and the ejaculatory
duct.

Testis biopsy

A needle sample is taken from the testis, or a tiny
snippet of tubules is taken at open operation (Fig.
23.3). The tissue is put immediately into Bouin's

Table 23.1 Klinefelter's syndrome.

Tall thin
Gynaecomastia
Small testes and penis
Elevated gonadotrophins and hyalinised testicular tubules

Table 23.2 Normal semen parameters.

Key features	
Colour	Grey–yellow
Volume	2.5 mL
Sperm density	20–200 million/mL
Motility	>50% at 4 hours
Abnormal forms	<50%
Fructose	Present

preservative fluid (not ordinary formalin) to avoid
distortion of the histology. It is rare for a testis
biopsy to show any condition that can be put right
by treatment.

Treatment

Azospermia

If the FSH and luteinizing hormone (LH) are elevated, testicular biopsy will add nothing to the
diagnosis. If the biopsy shows *maturation arrest*
(Fig. 23.4), completion of the cycle of spermatogenesis may be attempted by medical therapy. The
presence of *lymphocytes* in the biopsies suggests an
immunological problem.

Blockage to the seminal tract may occur from a
number of causes. There may have been exposure
to mercury in childhood, once a common component of 'teething powders' which paralysed the
microcilia in the bronchioles as well as in the epididymis. Congenital absence of vasa could occur. A
blockage in the vas deferens can be demonstrated
with a vasogram (Fig. 23.5) which may be treated
by epididymovasostomy (Fig. 23.6). A transrectal
ultrasound scan may show dilatation of the seminal vesicles, secondary to blockage of the ejaculatory ducts which may be relieved by transurethral
incision of the ejaculatory ducts.

Oligospermia

When a 'low sperm count' has been reported, the
first step must be to check it with a properly vali-
dated computerised technique. Because of the errors in the usual methods, claims that any form
of treatment has done good must be treated with
considerable scepticism. Loose pants and ice packs
have had their vogue. Operations on varicoceles,

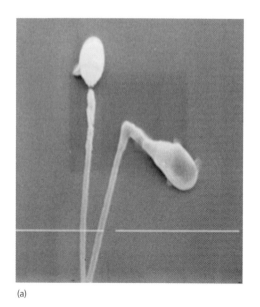

(a)

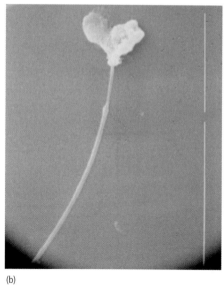

(b)

Figure 23.2 Scanning electron microscopy of 'abnormal' morphology of sperms.

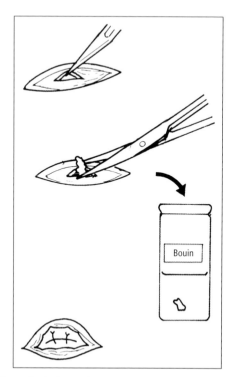

Figure 23.3 Biopsy of testis.

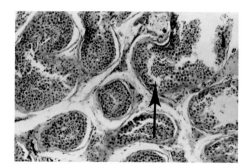

Figure 23.4 Maturation arrest: the arrow shows immature cells shed into the lumen of the tubule.

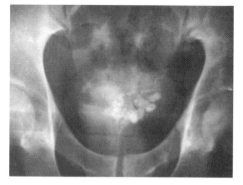

Figure 23.5 Vasogram showing filling of the vas deferens and seminal vesicle on the left side.

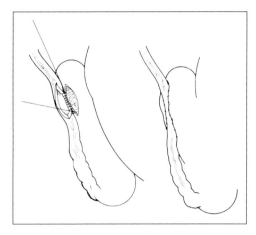

Figure 23.6 Epididymovasostomy.

whether they can be seen, or have to be detected by Doppler studies in symptomless men, should be regarded with even more scepticism. This is an area which cries out for 'evidence-based' decision making.

Vasectomy

Consent

Both partners must understand that vasectomy is likely to be irreversible. It must also be explained that however carefully the vasa are divided, the ends may join each other again. Usually this is detected within the first few months after the vasectomy (early failure) but in something like 1:2000 cases, it occurs some years later (late failure) and takes place irrespective of what type of operation has been done. Until all the sperms have disappeared from the ejaculate the couple must continue to use contraceptive precautions.

Because of the risk of medicolegal consequences, all these points should be fully discussed, and spelled out on the consent form.

Procedure

Vasectomy can be performed under local or general anaesthesia. When there has been previous surgery in the inguinal region or scrotum, general anaesthesia may be preferable.

The large number of different techniques described today shows that none of them is perfect. There is no objective evidence that any one method is superior to another in terms of preventing either early or late reunion.

Usually a small length of vas is removed, and the ends are treated to seal them off in the hope of preventing spontaneous reunion (Fig. 23.7). The ends may be ligated with absorbable or non-absorbable material or diathermised. Some surgeons seal one vas, others both. Some surgeons back one end, some both. Some stitch the sheath of the vas to interpose a layer of 'fascia' between the two ends. Many do not. Both early and late recurrence have been reported after all of these methods, and it almost certainly takes place more frequently than is generally appreciated: in 10% of one series of men who came up to have their vasectomy reversed it was found that spermatozoa were present in their pre-reversal specimens.

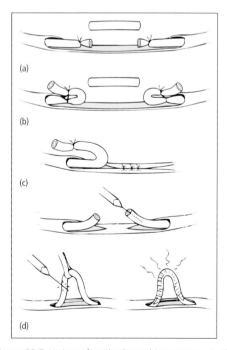

(a)

(b)

(c)

(d)

Figure 23.7 Variety of methods used in vasectomy in the hope of preventing early or late recanalisation.

Complications

1 Haematoma is common, from reactionary bleeding from small scrotal veins that go into spasm during the operation and escape notice. A large haematoma is dealt with by early evacuation of the clot and haemostasis. Small collections usually resolve spontaneously.

2 Infection may take place, usually at the site of a skin suture, sometimes in a haematoma.

3 Pain in the scrotum: A small number of patients continue to complain of pain in the scrotum for which no cause can be found.

4 Sperm granuloma: Sometimes a sperm granuloma is found at the site of the division of the vas or epididymis to give a typical tender nodular swelling.

'Reversal' of vasectomy: reanastomosis of the vas

The ends of the vas are found, trimmed back to the lumen, and sewn together (Fig. 23.8). Most

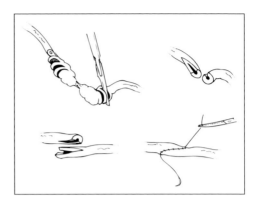

Figure 23.8 Reversal of vasectomy.

surgeons use magnification when performing this operation. Success in terms of sperms finding their way through the anastomosis can be expected in over 80%, but only about 50% will father children. There are many possible reasons for this, including the possible development of auto-antibodies during the time that sperms have been obstructed in the epididymis.

Chapter 24

Minimally invasive urology: laparoscopy and robotics

Surgery is a therapeutic approach adopted by surgeons to enter various cavities in the body to remedy various pathological ailments in the body. Incisions are needed to allow surgeons access into the necessary cavities and use their eyes and hands to carry out therapeutic manoeuvres. Advances and innovations gave surgeons the chance to change routes of access and offer significant improvements in surgical operative treatments performed under magnification. Although open surgery is still often necessary, minimally invasive surgery is being increasingly applied in various surgical fields.

Laparoscopy

Laparoscopy is a surgical procedure in which a fibre-optic instrument is inserted through the abdominal wall to view the organs in the abdomen and permit small-scale surgery.

Patient selection

Adequate history and physical examination are the cornerstones for patient selection for laparoscopy.

Contra-indications

- *Relative:* Prior abdominal and pelvic surgery, pelvic fibrosis, obesity, hiatus hernia, non-reducible herniations of the abdomen/inguinal hernia, umbilical abnormalities and abdominal aortic/iliac aneurysm.
- *Absolute:* Abdominal wall infections, generalised peritonitis, bowel obstruction and uncorrected coagulopathy.

Anaesthetics

The ideal anaesthetic technique should aim at maximal safety for the patient. The technique should provide adequate muscle relaxation and analgesia, and allow for rapid postoperative recovery. Laparoscopic procedures often need the Trendelenberg position and frequent alteration in the position of the operating table. Thus precautions to safeguard against the risk of peripheral neuropathy and protection of bony prominences by adequate padding and secure velcro strapping to the operating table. Laparoscopic surgery has been performed under local, regional and general anaesthesia. The technique chosen should be based on the medical condition of the patient, the indication for the procedure, the preference or choice of the patient and the surgeon's needs.

Lecture Notes: Urology, 6th edition. By John Blandy and Amir Kaisary. Published 2009 by Blackwell Publishing. ISBN: 978-1-4051-2270-2.

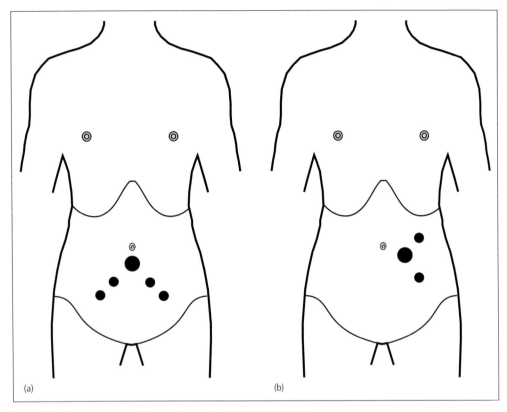

Figure 24.1 Trocar placement: (a) prostate surgery and (b) renal surgery.

Pneumoperitoneum

Insufflation of CO_2 aims at instilling approximately 3–6 L of CO_2 into the abdomen.

1 *Insufflator:* This is a piece of equipment which has a CO_2 gas cylinder attached to it and has an insufflation tube line to be attached to the patient. Dials indicate clearly the total CO_2 delivered, actual and set CO_2 flow rate, pressure set point and intra-abdominal pressure. A spare tank of CO_2 should always be available in the operating room.

2 *Trocars/ports:* A laparoscopic trocar is a means through which access into the abdomen is secured. All trocars have two common components: a sharp obturator to facilitate access into the abdominal cavity and a sheath through which the obturator passes. The sheath may have a side port for CO_2 insufflation. The sheath has a valve or a membrane through which instruments may be introduced without loss of CO_2 from the abdomen. Trocars are reusable or disposable. A primary trocar is the first trocar to be placed after a pneumoperitoneum is obtained. Secondary trocars follow. Sites for trocar placements are chosen to facilitate access to the organ to be operated upon (Fig. 24.1).

3 *Laparoscopic instruments:* A wide assortment facilitates all laparoscopic procedures. They are available in both re-usable and disposable types. Most standard laparoscopic instruments are available in diameters ranging from 3 to 12 mm and 35 cm in length. These diameters allow their passage through a given trocar and are of a sufficient length to reach the operative site. They include graspers, incising instruments, retractors, needle holders, knot pushers, specimen entrapment sacks and aspiration/irrigation devices. Surgical clips

and staplers have been adapted for use through the laparoscopy ports to secure/ligate vessels, close luminal structures and re-approximate tissue edges.

Improvements in design and material are continually being made laparoscopy equipments and instruments.

Complications of laparoscopy

These mainly fall into two main categories: intra-operative and postoperative groups.

1 Intraoperative: These are either associated with anaesthesia or related to laparoscopic technique.

  (a) Cardiovascular:
- *Gas embolus:* It can cause cardiovascular collapse. It is usually due to inadvertent placement of the insufflations needle into a blood vessel or vascular organ. When a large volume of gas reaches the right ventricle, an air lock impedes the pulmonary circulation. The consequent cascade of events may lead to a catastrophic right ventricular failure, drop in venous flow and left ventricular of output.
- *Hypotension:* Intra-peritoneal abdominal insufflation up to pressure of 20 mm Hg is well tolerated. However, intra-abdominal pressure more than 30 mm Hg may decrease the cardiac output and arterial blood pressure.
- *Hypertension:* Hypercapnia due to absorption of CO_2 may stimulate the sympathetic nervous system leading to tachycardia and hypertension. Patients with essential are vulnerable.
- *Arrhythmias:* Bradycardia, tachycardia and premature ventricular contractions could occur.

  (b) Pulmonary:
- *Hypoxaemia:* Ventilation–perfusion imbalance can be caused by a combination of the Trendelenburg position and the abdominal contents resting on the diaphragm. This can in turn lead to decreased lung volume, atelectasis and blood pooling in the dependent parts of the lungs.
- *Acidosis:* Absorption of insufflated CO_2 and ventilation–perfusion imbalance could lead to autonomous stimulation of the central nervous system. This may lead to acidosis, myocardial depression, vaso-dilatation and hypotension.
- *Aspiration:* Trendelenburg position and increased intra-abdominal pressure could put the anaesthetised patient at risk of regurgitation and aspiration of gastric contents.
- *Pneumothorax, pneumo-mediastinum and pneumo-pericardium:* These can occur if a trocar is placed above the 12th rib, or if there are presence of diaphragmatic defects or positive pressure trauma to the lings.

  (c) Miscellaneous:
- subcutaneous emphysema;
- vascular injuries range from haematoma formation in the abdominal wall to laceration of the abdominal aorta;
- perforation of a solid organ or a hollow viscous; and
- peripheral nerve damage.

2 Postoperative:

  (a) *Fever/peritonitis:* It may represent the first sign of a missed intra-operative bowel perforation or urinary leakage.

  (b) *Delayed haemorrhage:* It could be one of the causes of postoperative haemodynamic instability.

  (c) *Incisional hernia:* Risk of abdominal contents herniation via a small diameter trocar (≤ 5 mm) is low but could occur via a trocar ≥ 10 mm site.

  (d) *Impaired renal functions:* It could be secondary to intra-operative unrecognised bladder perforation or urinary leakage.

Establishing a well-trained laparoscopy team with an experienced surgical assistant and a scrub nurse is a must. The role played by an attentive anaesthetic team cannot be overestimated. Meticulous attention to details is essential to success in successful laparoscopy procedures.

Robotics

Robotics is a branch of technology concerned with the design, construction, operation and application of robots. A robot is a mechanical device that can perform pre-programmed repetitive tasks creating a 'Master–Slave' system. In industry, robots are used for mass production and improved efficiency. Advances in the field led to the creation of robotic integrated surgical systems which can assist surgeons in performing surgical procedures in real time with improved vision and surgical precision. It allows computer-assisted control of laparoscopic instruments with enhanced degree of manoeuvrability and stereoscopic vision. A range of surgical procedures including cardiac bypass surgery, mitral valve repair, hernia repair, hysterectomy and other procedures are examples of a growing list. In urology, prostatectomy for early prostate cancer was

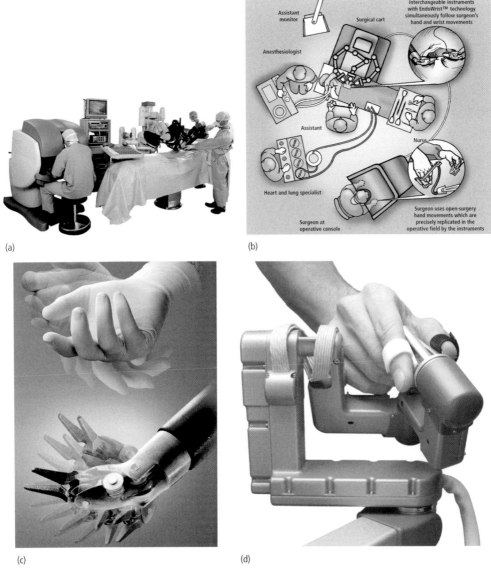

Figure 24.2 da Vinci Robot: (a) system; (b) theatre layout; (c) EndoWrist; (d) hand control; and (e) operator view. Photos courtesy of Intuitive Surgical, Inc., 2008.

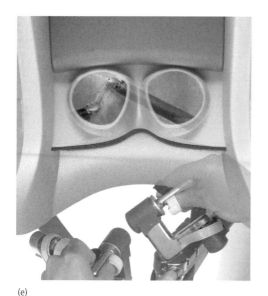

(e)

Figure 24.2 (*Continued*)

probably the first attractive urological procedure to attract application of robotic-assisted surgery. The da Vinci Surgical System (Fig. 24.2) offers 10x operative magnification allowing for more precise surgical performance and subsequently improving outcomes relating to sexual function and continence. Less likely requirement for blood transfusion, less postoperative pain, faster recovery times and equivalent cancer outcome control are expected advantages. Outcome data on robotic versus traditional surgery are becoming increasingly recognised. It is also expensive. Thus opinion on the future of robotic surgery remains divided among surgeons despite the growing list of various urological procedures performed with robotic assistance.

Self-assessment MCQs

1. A 27-year-old man is shot in the left flank. IVP shows extravasation of contrast just below the ureteropelvic junction. On CT scan, the spleen and bowel appear to be uninvolved. The next step in management is:
   a. emergency arteriogram
   b. percutaneous nephrostomy
   c. percutaneous nephrostomy and antegrade catheter
   d. explore the injury transabdominally
   e. explore the injury through the flank

2. A girl of 14 is kicked by her horse and suffers a rupture of her kidney. Correct initial management is likely to be:
   a. resuscitation followed by cystoscopy and retrograde ureterography as soon as stable
   b. renal arteriography followed by immediate exploration
   c. resuscitation, intravenous urography and initial observation in ITU
   d. renal ultrasound and percutaneous nephrostomy drainage of the kidney
   e. immediate exploration of the kidney

3. Theories of urinary stone formation include the following:
   a. sub-epithelial Randall's plaque
   b. renal hypersecretion of stone-forming salts
   c. primary hypoparathyroidism
   d. renal tubular acidosis
   e. immobilisation

4. A 61-year-old man with a history of stone disease and multiple bilateral ureterolithotomies is seen with a fever of 103°F, pyuria and microheamaturia. An IVP reveals a 6-mm right mid-ureteral calculus with delayed function of the right kidney and marked obstruction. In addition to beginning parenteral antibiotics, the most reasonable immediate management option is:
   a. emergency ESWL
   b. placement of a ureteral stent to bypass the obstruction
   c. percutaneous nephrostomy and antegrade basketing of the calculus under fluoroscopy
   d. ureteroscopic stone extraction
   e. emergency ureterolithotomy

5. Renal calculi could contain the following except:
   a. cholesterol
   b. oxalate
   c. phosphate
   d. urate
   e. cysteine

6. The major cause of uric acid stone formation in patients with ileostomy is:
   a. dehydration
   b. hyperuricemia
   c. low urinary pH
   d. hyperurucosuria
   e. malabsorption

7. A previously fit young woman of 28 years presents with acute loin pain and a fever. An emergency IVU shows a right hydronephrosis with obstruction of the right ureter caused by a 10-mm stone impacted in

the right ureter at the level of a sacroiliac joint. The most appropriate immediate treatment will be:

a. MSU, antibiotics and observe for 48 hours before any further intervention
b. immediate percutaneous nephrostomy
c. immediate cystoscopy and the passage of a ureteric catheter by-passed the stone to relieve the obstruction
d. immediate operation with endoscopic ureteroscopy and destruction of the stone with endoscopic removal of fragments
e. analgesia and a forced diuresis

8. Complications of shock wave lithotripsy of a renal stone include:
a. haematuria
b. sub-capsular haematoma
c. ureteric obstruction by stone fragments
d. significant loin brushing
e. all of the above

9. Metabolic causes of renal stone formation include all the following except:
a. hypercalcuria
b. cystinuria
c. renal tubular acidosis
d. myxoedema
e. hyperoxaluria

10. Bladder stones have been associated with:
a. squamous carcinoma of the urothelium
b. non-absorbable sutures in the bladder
c. obstructive large prostate hypertrophy
d. strangury
e. all of the above

11. In renal cell carcinoma, stage III indicates:
a. tumour limited to renal capsule
b. lung metastases
c. regional lymph node involvement
d. none of the above
e. all of the above

12. A 71-year-old man has sudden, dull, right flank pain, nausea and gross haematuria. KUB shows no significant calcification. IVP shows non-function of the right kidney with developing dense nephrogram effect at six hours. The next step should be:

a. CT scan
b. renal scan
c. renal aniography
d. renal ultrasound
e. retrograde pyelogram

13. Possible symptoms/findings of a patient with a renal parenchymal carcinoma could include:
a. a renal mass
b. haematuria
c. intermittent fevers
d. erythrocytosis
e. all of the above

14. Aetiology of urethelial carcinoma includes exposure to the following possible carcinogens or related conditions except:
a. aniline dyes
b. tobacco
c. schistosomiasis
d. alcohol
e. leukoplakia of the urothelium

15. Intravesical therapy in management of an advanced bladder carcinoma (T4) include the following:
a. Epodil
b. BCG
c. Mitomycin-C
d. Adriamycin
e. none of the above

16. Stage T2 transitional cell carcinoma of the bladder indicates:
a. a non-invasive lesion unto the suburothelial tissue
b. deep infiltration into the muscle; a mobile mass
c. a fixed mass
d. superficial infiltration into the muscle; ill-defined thickening on bimanual examination
e. carcinoma in situ

17. Transitional cell carcinoma of the ureter is most frequently associated with:
    a. chronic pyelonephritis
    b. recurrent renal stones
    c. cigarette smoking
    d. chronic aspirin ingestion
    e. Balkan ancestry

18. Valuable routine investigations of painless haematuria include:
    a. urine cystology
    b. intravenous urography (IVU)
    c. cysto-urethroscopy
    d. all of the above
    e. none of the above

19. Painless haematuria in a male patient aged 78 years could be due to all the following except:
    a. renal cell carcinoma
    b. bladder carcinoma
    c. seminoma
    d. ureteric carcinoma

20. Bimanual examination of the bladder under general anaesthetic in a case of T2 bladder carcinoma would be:
    a. no abnormality
    b. a well-defined fixed mass
    c. an ill-defined localised thickening
    d. a well-defined mobile mass
    e. an ill-defined fixed mass

21. Urinary diversion metabolic complication is:
    a. hypernatimic alkalosis
    b. hypercholaraemic acidosis
    c. hypercapnic alkalosis
    d. renal metabolic acidosis

22. The following drugs can sometimes precipitate retention of urine in men with symptoms of bladder outlet obstruction:
    a. Sudafed
    b. Oxybutynin hydrochloride
    c. Tricyclic anti-depressants
    d. Carbachol
    e. Cimetidine

23. The prostate contains the highest organ concentration of which of the following:
    a. magnesium
    b. cholesterol
    c. urokinase
    d. citric acid
    e. zinc

24. In men with benign prostatic hyperplasia, the symptoms which correlate most with obstruction are all the following except:
    a. nocturia
    b. urgency
    c. frequency
    d. slow stream
    e. terminal dribbling

25. A man of 60 is investigated for symptoms of bladder outlet obstruction and the diagnosis is made of moderate benign prostatic hypertrophy leading to an obstructed urinary flow and incomplete bladder emptying. It is decided to treat him conservatively with medication. He is on no other medication and is otherwise fit. Appropriate drugs would include:
    a. terazosin (Hytrin)
    b. prazosin (Hypovase)
    c. tamsulosin (Flomax)
    d. finasteride
    e. all of the above

26. A 65-year-old man has continuous urinary dribbling following a trans-urethral resection of the prostate for benign hyperplasia. Possible explanations include:
    a. chronic retention of urine
    b. damage to the sphincter mechanism
    c. urinary tract infection
    d. gross detrusor instability
    e. all of the above

27. Complications of prostatectomy include:
    a. clot retention
    b. urethritis and stricture
    c. infertility
    d. osteitis pubis
    e. all of the above

28. Chronic urine retention in prostatic hypertrophy is:
  a. painful
  b. painless
  c. intermittently painful
  d. continuously painful
  e. occasionally painless

29. Hormonal management of metastatic prostatic carcinoma include:
  a. bilateral orchidectomy
  b. oestrogen
  c. LHRH agonists
  d. LHRH antagonist
  e. all of the above

30. The most frequent site of distant metastases in prostates carcinoma is:
  a. lungs
  b. lymph nodes
  c. liver
  d. bones
  e. brain

31. Prostatic-specific antigen appears to be most accurate in:
  a. differentiating carcinoma from benign hyperplasia of the prostate
  b. predicting residual disease post-radical prostatectomy
  c. predicting stage of carcinoma of the prostate
  d. predicting elevations of acid phosphatase
  e. predicting urinary obstruction

32. A 75-year-old man has a well-differentiated (Gleason 2 + 1) adenocarcinoma in 2 of 88 chips of a trans-urethral prostatectomy (TURP) specimen. All chips were examined. The most appropriate management is:
  a. periodic rectal examination and PSA measurement
  b. immediate repeat TURP
  c. immediate repeat TURP plus needle biopsy
  d. repeat TURP in three months
  e. repeat TURP plus needle biopsy in three months

33. Complications of urethral stricture include:
  a. periurethral abscess
  b. urethral diverticulum
  c. urine extravasation
  d. all of the above
  e. none of the above

34. A urethral stricture may develop in men as a consequence of:
  a. an indwelling catheter
  b. gonocaccal urethritis
  c. syphilis
  d. urethral trauma
  e. all of the above

35. The single most important sign of urethral injury after pelvic trauma is:
  a. pelvic fracture
  b. blood in the urethral meatus
  c. inability to void
  d. haematuria
  e. pelvic haematoma

36. The most frequent complication of rupture of the prostatomembranous urethra is:
  a. impotence
  b. incontinence
  c. abscess
  d. fistula
  e. stricture

37. A fall stride injury could be associated with
  a. rupture of the bulbar urethra
  b. rupture of the posterior urethra
  c. a risk of subsequent stricture
  d. none of the above
  e. all of the above

38. Klinefelter's syndrome includes the following criteria:
  a. tall and thin
  b. small testes and penis
  c. elevated gonadotrophins
  d. hyalinised testicular tubules
  e. all of the above

39. Normal semen parameters include all the following except:
   a. colour: grey–yellow
   b. volume: 2.5 mL
   c. sperm density: 20–200 million/mL
   d. motility: >50% at 4 hours
   e. abnormal forms: < 50%
   f. fructose: absent

40. Carcinoma of the penis is:
   a. squamous cell type
   b. transitional cell type
   c. glandular adenocarcinoma
   d. basal cell type
   e. small cell carcinoma

41. The most frequent testicular tumour is:
   a. seminoma
   b. teratoma
   c. lymphoma
   d. interstitial tumour of Leydig
   e. lipoma

42. A 29-year-old man was seen by a dermatologist for a lesion of the glans penis. A shave biopsy was performed which revealed squamous cell carcinoma in situ. Physical examination shows a well-healed scar and no inguinal adenopathy. The next step in management should be:
   a. simple penectomy
   b. laser fulgration of the lesion
   c. excision of previous scar
   d. total penectomy with biopsy of sentinel nodes
   e. observation only

43. A 9-year-old boy is referred with an enlarged left side of the scrotum approximately for 15-hour duration. The boy noted mild discomfort in the scrotum following a football rugby game. The discomfort progressed during the night and prevented him from sleeping. A 6-year-old sister had mumps one month ago. The left side of the scrotum was markedly enlarged and slightly erythematous. The scrotum was diffusely tender without localisation. His temperature was 100°F and white blood cell count was 8,400 with a normal differential. Urine analysis was normal. The most likely diagnosis is:
   a. acute epididymitis
   b. torsion of the spermatic cord
   c. mumps orchitis
   d. traumatic haematocoele
   e. incarcerated inguinal hernia

44. The major complication from long-term oral androgenic agents in the treatment of impotence is:
   a. development of benign enlargement of the prostate
   b. gynaecomastia
   c. hepatotoxicity
   d. weight gain
   e. infertility

45. Common causes of azospermia include:
   a. previous syphilitic infection
   b. previous gonorrhoeal infection
   c. vasa aplasia
   d. epididymal cyst
   e. all of the above

46. In an 8-year-old boy with retractile testis, the best management would be:
   a. periodic re-examination
   b. no further follow up
   c. orchidopexy
   d. LHRH agonist
   e. HCG

47. A 20-year-old man with a 2-cm palpable area of induration on the left testicle. Ultrasonography reveals a non-homogenous, well-circumscribed, intratesticular mass. The best course of management is:
   a. observation and serial ultrasonography
   b. surgical exploration
   c. ultrasound guided needle biopsy of the testicular mass
   d. repeat ultrasonography with coloured Doppler scanning
   e. none of the above

48. The obliterated umbilical artery originates from which of the following arteries:
a. superior gluteal artery
b. obturator artery
c. middle sacral artery
d. internal iliac artery
e. external iliac artery

49. True priapism:
a. usually resolves spontaneously
b. may result in a pulmonary embolus
c. is most commonly the outcome of trauma
d. usually involves the corpus cavernosum
e. may result in fibrosis of the corpus spongiosum

50. A 27-year-old man developed sudden onset of pain in the penis during vigorous sexual intercourse. He heard a "pop" sound which was followed by a swelling of the penis, ecchymosis and distortion of the right side of the penis at mid-shaft. An urethrogram performed was normal. The preferred management plan should be:
a. suprapubic catheter and pressure dressing of penile shaft
b. Foley urethral catheter and ice pack
c. pressure dressing and allow home for review after 48 hours
d. exploration and repair of the corpora
e. ice pack and delayed exploration if the swelling persists

Answers to MCQs

1. b	**18.** d	**35.** b
2. c	**19.** c	**36.** e
3. b	**20.** c	**37.** e
4. b	**21.** d	**38.** e
5. b–e	**22.** b	**39.** f
6. e	**23.** x	**40.** a
7. c	**24.** b	**41.** a
8. e	**25.** e	**42.** b
9. d	**26.** e	**43.** c
10. e	**27.** e	**44.** a
11. d	**28.** b	**45.** c
12. a	**29.** e	**46.** a
13. e	**30.** d	**47.** b
14. d	**31.** b	**48.** d
15. e	**32.** a	**49.** d
16. d	**33.** d	**50.** d
17. c	**34.** e	

Glossary

agenesis: Greek α plus γε'νεσις (creation)

albumen: Latin, egg-white

allantois: Greek αλλας (sausage)

Alport, Cecil (1880–1959): South African physician

ampulla: Latin, a flask

aplasia: Greek α plus πλασσειν (to form)

balanitis: Greek βαλανος (the glans penis)

Barr, Murray (1908): Contemporary Canadian anatomist

Behçet, Hulúsi (1889–1948): Turkish dermatologist

Bellini, Lorenzo (1643–1704): Anatomist of Pisa

Bence-Jones, Henry (1814–73): Physician, London

Benedict, Stanley Rossiter (1884–1936): Biochemist, New York

Bertin, Exupère Joseph (1712–81): Associate anatomist, Academy of Sciences, Paris

Bilharz, Theodor Maximilian (1825–62): German physician working in Cairo who discovered *Schistosoma haematobium*

Boari, Achille (b. 1894): Italian urologist

Bonney, W.F. Victor (1872–1953): Gynaecologist, Middlesex Hospital, London

bougie: French, candle (the best wax came from Bujiyah in Algeria)

Bouin, Paul (1870–1962): Histologist of Strasbourg: devised fixative containing picric and acetic acids as well as formalin

Bowman, Sir William (1816–92): Ophthalmic surgeon, London

Brucella: Microorganisms discovered by Sir William Bruce (1855–1931), British surgeon

Buck, Gordon (1807–77): Surgeon, New York

Burch, J.C: American gynaecologist

Buschke, Abraham (1868–1943): German pathologist

calix. Greek κα'λιξ (cup). Often confused with Graeco-Latin κα'λυξ (the leaves covering the bud of a flower), and incorrectly written as calyx

Camper, Peter (1772–89): Physician of Amsterdam

cannula: Latin (canna, a reed)

catheter: Greek καθετηρ, καθεμη (to send down)

Chlamydia: Greek χλα'μυς (cloak)

chordée: Painful curvature of the penis: French *cordée*

clitoris: Greek (κλειτορι'ς)

Colles, Abraham (1773–1843): Professor of Surgery in Dublin

Conn, Jerome W. (1907): American physician

Cowper, William (1666–1709): Surgeon of London

creatinine: Greek κρε'ας (flesh: product of catabolism of protein)

Crohn, Burrill B. (1884–1983): Gastroenterologist, New York

Cushing, Harvey (1869–1939): Neurosurgeon of Boston

de la Peyronie, François (1678–1747): Surgeon of Paris

Denonvilliers, Charles Pierre (1802–72): Surgeon of Paris

detrusor: Latin (detrudere, to push down)

diabetes: Latin (syphon)

dilate: Latin, dilatare: *di-* plus *latus* (wide) hence dilatation (dilation is incorrect)

Doppler, Christian Johann (1803–53): Austrian physicist

Ducrey, Augusto (1860–1940): Dermatologist of Rome

Dupuytren, Baron Guillaume (1777–1835): French surgeon and pathologist

dysplasia: Greek δυς (difficult, bad etc.) plus πλασσειν (formation)

Echinococcus: Greek ε'χι⁻νος (hedgehog), κο'κκος (grain, seed)

ectopic. Greek εκτω'πος (displaced)

enuresis: Greek ε'νουρειν (incontinence): usually applied today to bed-wetting

epididymis: Greek ε'πι plus διδυμοι (twins – testes)

epispadias: Greek ε'πι plus σπα'δον (a rent or tear)

Escherich, Theodor (1857–1911): Paediatrician of Munich

exstrophy: Greek ε'ξστρεφειν (to turn inside out)

Falloppius, Gabriel (1523–62): Anatomist of Padua: favourite pupil of Vesalius

fasciculata: Latin *fasciculus* (packet, bundle)

Foley, Frederic Eugene Basil (1891–1966): Urologist of Minneapolis–St Paul

fossa: Latin (ditch)

fraenum, fraenulum: Latin (bridle)

fundus: Bottom

Ghoneim, Mohamed: Egyptian urologist of Mansoura

Gimbernat, Don Manuel Louis (1734–1816): Anatomist, Barcelona

Giraldes, Joachim (1808–75): Professor of Surgery, Paris

Gleason, D.F: Pathologist of Minneapolis St Pauls, USA

glomerulus: Latin (little ball)

Goodpasture, Ernest William (1886–1960): American pathologist

Grawitz, Paul Albert (1850–1932): Pathologist of Greifswald

gubernaculum: Latin (rudder; described by John Hunter, sometimes called Hunter's gubernaculum)

Hartnup: Surname of English family in whom the disease was first described

Henle, Freidrich (1809–85): Anatomist of Berlin

Henoch, E. (1820–1910): Paediatrician, Berlin

hilum: Latin (eye of seed or bean, hence applied to kidney)

Hounsfield, Sir Godfrey Newbold (1919–2004): Nobel laureate, inventor of CT and MRI scanners

Hunner, Guy Leroy (1868–1951): Gynaecologist, Johns Hopkins, Baltimore

hyaline: Greek υ'αλου (glass)

hydatid: Greek υ'δωρ (drop of water)

hydrocele: Greek υδωρ (water) plus κη'λη (swelling; often misspelt hydrocoele from confusion with κο'ιλιακος meaning belly)

insipidus: Latin (tasteless; diabetes insipidus, the urine does not taste sweet)

Jaboulay, Mathieu (1860–1913): Surgeon of Lyons

Jensen, Carl Oluf (1864–1934): Pathologist of Copenhagen

Katayama, Kunika (1886–1931): Japanese Physician

Klinefelter, Harry Fitch (b. 1912): Contemporary radiologist, Massachusetts General Hospital

Leydig, Franz von (1821–1908): Anatomist of Bonn

litho-: Greek λιθος (stone), hence tripsy, from τριβειν (to crush), τομη' (cut), λα'παξειν (to evacuate)

Littré, Alexis (1658–1726): Anatomist of Paris

Löwenstein, Ernst pathologist of Vienna

malacoplakia: Greek μαλακο'ς and πλακος (plaque)

Marshall, Victor F. (1913–1996): Urologist, New York Memorial Hospital

meatus: Latin (passage or channel)

mellitus: Latin *mel* (honey, honey-sweet; diabetes mellitus, urine tastes sweet)

micturition: Latin (urinate), derived from *mingere* (to mix). Originally meant frequency

Millin, Terence (1903–1980): Irish urologist working in London

Morgagni, Giovanni Battista (1682–1771): Anatomist of Padua

Müller, Johannes (1801–58): Physiologist of Berlin

navicularis: Latin (shaped like a boat)

Neisser, Albert Ludwig Siegmund (1855–1916): Dermatologist, Breslau

nephro-: Greek νε'φρον. Nephrosis, -οσις (condition), nephritis, -ητις (inflammation)

nexus: Latin (tying together, as in connect etc.)

nocturia: Latin *nocte* (night: passing abnormal amounts of urine in the night)

Page, I. Harriet Contemporary American physician, Cleveland clinic

pampiniform: Latin *pampinus* (tendril)

Papanicolaou, George N. (1883–1962): Greek pathologist working in New York

papilla: Latin (nipple)

papilloma: Latin (nipple) plus Greek ωμα (tumour)

Petit, Jean Louis (1674–1760): Parisian surgeon, elected to the Royal Society of London

Pfannenstiel, Hermann Johann (1862–1909): Gynaecologist, Breslau

polyuria: Greek πο'λυ (much) plus ο'υρια (passing much urine)

posthitis: Greek πο'σθε (foreskin)

Potter, Edith Louise (b. 1901): American perinatal pathologist

Queyrat, L. (b. 1911): Dermatologist, Paris

Randall, Alexander (1883–1930): Urologist, Philadelphia

Raz, Shlomo Contemporary American urologist, UCLA

Rehn, Ludwig (1849–1930): Surgeon, Frankfurt

reticularis: Latin (net-like)

Rovsing, N.T. (1862–1927): Professor of Surgery, Copenhagen

Sachse, Hans Contemporary German urologist

Scarpa, Antonio (1747–1832): Anatomist, Pavia

Schistosoma: Greek σχιστω (split) plus σωμα (body)

Schönlein, Johann L. (1793–1864): German physician

Scott, F. Brantley Contemporary American urologist

Scribner, Belding H. (b. 1921): Contemporary American nephrologist

Sertoli, Enrico (1842–1910): Anatomist, Pavia

Shy–Drager, Milton G. Shy (1919–1967), Glen A. Drager (b. 1917): American neurologists

spermatozoa: Greek σπερμα (seed) plus ζωιον (animal)

Stamey, Thomas A. Contemporary American Urologist, Stanford, California

strangury: Greek στρα'γξ (drop squeezed out) plus ουπον (slow and painful urination)

teratoma: Greek τε'ρας (monster) plus ομα (swelling)

testis: Latin (witness)

Treponema. Greek τρεπειν (turn), νεμα (thread)

Trichomonas: Greek θριξ (hair) plus μονος (one; though it has three to five hairs)

trocar: French *trois carrés* (three sharp edges)

urethra: Greek ουρηθρα

utriculus: Latin (small bag)

varicocele: Latin *varus* (bent) plus Greek κη'λη (swelling)

vas: Latin (a vessel)

verumontanum: Latin *veru* (a spit) *montanum* (mountainous)

vesicle: Latin (a little bladder)

von Brunn, A. (1841–95): Professor of Anatomy, Gottingen

von Fehling, Hermann Christian (1812–85): German chemist

vulva: Latin (a wrapper)

Whitaker, Robert H. (b. 1939): Contemporary urologist and anatomist, Cambridge

Wilms, Max (1867–1918): Surgeon, Heidelberg (nephroblastoma had previously been described by Rance in 1814)

Wolff, Kaspar Friedrich (1733–94): German anatomist, working in St Petersburg

xanthogranuloma: Greek ξανθο'ς (yellow)

Index